CREATING A

JUST

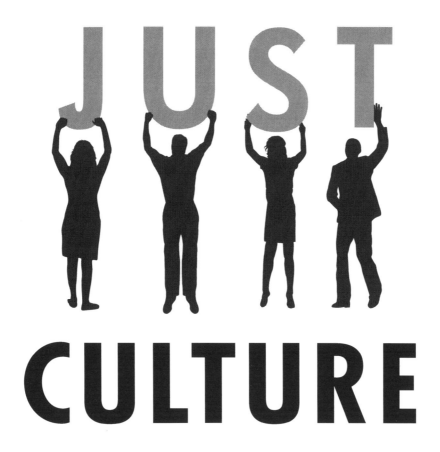

CULTURE

A Nurse Leader's Guide

VIVIAN B. MILLER, BA, CPHQ, LHRM, CPHRM, FASHRM
REVIEWED BY TERRY L. JONES, RN, PhD

HCPro

Creating a Just Culture: A Nurse Leader's Guide is published by HCPro, Inc.

Download the additional materials for this book at *www.hcpro.com/downloads/8752*.

ISBN: 978-1-60146-765-2

Vivian B. Miller, Author
Terry L. Jones, Author
Tami Swartz, Managing Editor
Michael Briddon, Executive Editor
Emily Sheahan, Group Publisher
Mike Mirabello, Senior Graphic Artist
Amanda Donaldson, Copyeditor
Sada Preisch, Proofreader
Matt Sharpe, Production Supervisor
Susan Darbyshire, Art Director
Jean St. Pierre, Senior Director of Operations

Advice given is general. Readers should consult professional counsel for specific legal, ethical, or clinical questions. Arrangements can be made for quantity discounts. For more information, contact:

HCPro, Inc.
75 Sylvan Street, Suite A-101
Danvers, MA 01923
Telephone: 800/650-6787 or 781/639-1872
Fax: 800/639-8511
E-mail: *customerservice@hcpro.com*

Visit HCPro online at: *www.hcpro.com* and *www.hcmarketplace.com*

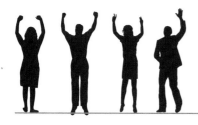

Contents

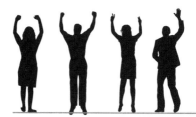

Dedication

To my dad, Jack Barker, who has supported me since the day I was born, who taught me to be responsible for my own actions, has always loved me, no questions asked, whether I was right or wrong, good or bad. His continuous pride in me has always made me want to do my very best.

To my parents-in-law, Jack and Jennie Miller, who embraced me as their daughter from the minute I married their son, who were as proud of me as any parents could be of their child, and who I have been very blessed to have as an integral part of my family.

To my husband, Mike Miller, who has loved me since I was 15 years old. You are honorable and hardworking, encouraging and supportive of every educational and professional move I have ever made, and you are also a terrific father to our two sons. Know that I love you very much, and will be forever grateful you stayed.

Lastly, to our sons, David and Sean: Having you in our lives made our house a home. Your father and I like to think we did a pretty good job where you are concerned—we did our best to give you everything you needed and much of what you wanted, while at the same time, trying to teach you that you have to work for what you want and that there are consequences associated with every action taken. We thank the stars every day that you turned out to be strong, educated, self-sufficient, independent, and family-oriented. We are so proud of you both and we love you very much.

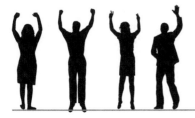

Preface

When I first began my career as the risk manager in a community hospital more than 20 years ago, incident reports were completed whenever there was a patient fall or a medication error or some other mistake that just couldn't be overlooked or ignored. The action taken most often documented by the unit manager or supervisor was that the employee involved was counseled. This traditional "blame and shame" punitive approach has always bothered me, particularly when I knew that the staff member, regardless of whether he or she was responsible for the occurrence, was absolutely doing the right thing by reporting the mistake, which was, by definition, an unusual event. This event was not ordinarily part of the routine course of his or her day. He or she reported the event to let risk management know of a potential exposure.

However, what the reporter usually got in return was disciplinary action. As a former clinician myself, I knew then, and the same is still true now even after all these years, that errors are made by people just like me—hardworking, educated folks who, for whatever reason, committed the error unintentionally without any anticipation of an adverse patient outcome, which usually occurs within the space of a just a few short minutes. The error usually occurs because of system flaws, such as the need to multitask, or to do a "work-around" from an established policy that is no longer reflective of current practice. Most of the time, there is no harm and no foul, but on occasion, the error can result in irreparable harm, not only to the patient and the patient's family, but also to the individual provider found responsible for the error.

I saw this firsthand when I managed the liability claims made against our hospital and providers. It was gut-wrenching to watch plaintiffs' counsel portray us as being insensitive and careless, and that

 Creating a Just Culture

as a result of this carelessness and deliberate inattentiveness to detail, the patient was injured. They would argue that the hospital and the provider should pay for their sins.

That is why, to me, embracing and supporting a just culture means taking the more appropriate approach to managing errors. Although I have seen a positive shift toward a more nonpunitive approach, I have to admit that I am acutely aware that this change can be a slow process. In most instances, the change does not take place overnight. I cannot just make a wish and snap my fingers in the hopes that the light will suddenly come on and every healthcare provider will "get it—" in other words, that each one will understand and appreciate the need to change our focus from being not only technically skilled, but also to being more patient-oriented when providing care, and more analytical about why errors occur rather than asking the question, "Who did it?" But I can say that I do believe that these last 11 years since the Institute of Medicine published its famous report on patient safety, *To Err Is Human: Building a Safer Health System*, there has been a growing awareness of the need to:

- Be more collaborative with the entire team of professionals providing care to our patients

- Be more open, honest, and communicative with our patients and their families

- More effectively manage the error reporting process in a way that will more justly and fairly hold staff accountable for their actions while, at the same time, improve processes that will prevent errors from occurring in the first place

At the end of his latest book entitled *Whack-a-Mole: The Price We Pay for Expecting Perfection*, David Marx says: "We have it within our control to build a safer, more compassionate society. While we can't expect perfection, we can hold each other accountable for the quality of our choices."[1]

I honestly believe that this is true. We are perfectly capable of and can successfully carry out those three goals bulleted above. Rather than punish the individual(s) involved with making the error, we can, and should, fairly and compassionately work with the individual by holding him or her responsible for the action while, at the same time, find out why the error occurred. Changes should be developed and implemented to correct the defective process and we should continuously monitor the effectiveness of these changes. If we can do this, then we will be doing what we set out to do when we chose healthcare as our profession in the first place: Continuously striving to provide consistently safe, skillful, high-quality patient care in a kind and professional manner.

There isn't a healthcare professional I know who has never made a medical mistake. As human beings, we are not perfect, and mistakes happen. Although hopefully not often, there may be a resulting adverse outcome, but as long as we know in our heart of hearts that every effort was made to put the patient's safety first—that we did the best we could to follow good policy and protocol and share our experiences with others without fear of reprisals so that improvements in processes can be made—then I can live with myself, and I believe others would agree.

There are several people, knowingly and unknowingly, who have influenced me as I have traveled down my professional road over the last 30 years, providing encouragement and advice, supporting my need to stay true to my work ethics and beliefs while, at the same time, teaching (or at least trying to teach) me to be patient and to listen to both sides before coming to any conclusions. These folks are:

Joann Rowell   William Minogue, MD

James R. Walker   Vahe Kazandjian

Karen E. Olscamp

Linda C. Jaecks

And for the rest of my family, friends, colleagues, and peers, thank you for being there whenever I asked or needed you to be there for me. Your support has always been, and will continue to be, most appreciated.

Vivian B. Miller, BA, CPHQ, LHRM, CPHRM, FASHRM

Reference

1. Marx, David. *Whack-a-Mole: The Price We Pay for Expecting Perfection.* By Your Side Studios, 2009.

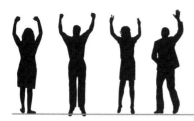

About the Authors

Vivian B. Miller, BA, CPHQ, LHRM, CPHRM, FASHRM

Vivian B. Miller, BA, CPHQ, LHRM, CPHRM, FASHRM, has more than 25 years of progressive consultative and managerial experience in professional liability claims, patient safety, quality, and risk management services within the insurance and healthcare delivery industries.

Miller is senior risk management specialist for the American Society for Healthcare Risk Management (ASHRM), serving as the internal staff resource on healthcare management content. Her personal knowledge, research and a professional network enhances the range and quality of ASHRM offerings. She identifies and develops risk management content to use as the basis for ASHRM programs, products and services; serves as an internal content consultant in the development of strategy initiatives, educational programs, communications campaigns, and other products and services, leading advocacy efforts; and serves as a risk management content resource to members and other constituents.

Miller is the former director of risk prevention for the University of Maryland Medical System (UMMS). Based in Baltimore, MD, the system is composed of corporate offices, an academic medical center, three specialty hospitals, five community hospitals; and is affiliated with three other community hospitals; and partners with the University of Maryland Schools of Medicine, Nursing, Pharmacy, and Dental Surgery, as well as offers specialty services to its community through its extensive physician network. Miller oversaw the risk prevention activities at the corporate level of the organization.

Prior to coming to UMMS, Miller was the research project manager and patient safety specialist for the Center for Performance Sciences, a research and consulting subsidiary of the Maryland Hospital Association, providing oversight for the Maryland Patient Safety Center's online, Web-based Adverse Event Reporting System offered to Maryland healthcare organizations as a way to collect and analyze data on adverse events and near misses. Prior to that, Miller has worked as a director of risk management in several acute care hospitals in the Baltimore–Washington, DC, metropolitan area. She obtained her Bachelor of Arts degree in Health Science and Policy from the University of Maryland, Baltimore County, in 1991 and is currently enrolled at the University of Maryland University College in the Master of Health Administration program. Miller is certified as a Professional in Healthcare Quality as well as in Risk Management, is a licensed risk manager in the state of Florida, and is a Fellow of the American Society for Healthcare Risk Management. She is an active member of the Maryland Society for Healthcare Risk Management, currently serving as treasurer; is chairperson of the American Society for Healthcare Risk Management's Foundation 2030 Fund; an active member of the National Association of Female Executives; and is listed in Manchester's Who's Who of Female Professionals.

Miller has written several articles and presented on numerous occasions on various patient safety and risk management topics.

Terry L. Jones, RN, PhD

Terry L. Jones, RN, PhD, is an assistant professor of nursing in the Department of Nursing Administration and Healthcare Systems at the University of Texas at Austin School of Nursing. Jones previously served as director of care management and interim vice president of nursing administration and chief nursing officer at Parkland Health & Hospital System in Dallas. She has been published nationally and has also presented nationally on various nursing topics.

Jones has been a registered nurse for more than 25 years.

       Creating a Just Culture

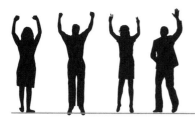

Introduction

This handbook serves as a guide for healthcare organizations that are ready to shift to an organizational culture dedicated to incorporating a strategic patient safety program that will balance accountability with safety and performance improvement. An organization's culture is what drives behavior, which in turn drives outcomes; in other words, if the organization as a whole (including the board, senior leadership, and medical staff) has embraced a culture that encourages adverse-event reporting without punitive consequences, while at the same time requiring the assumption of responsibility when an adverse event has occurred, the end result is what is known as a "just culture."

This is a concept that reconciles professional accountability with the need to create a safe environment in which individuals are not afraid to report medical errors. This handbook provides healthcare organizations with a hands-on approach toward designing safe systems that reduce the potential for patient harm, promote safe behavior, and encourage adverse-event reporting, which in turn will ultimately lead to a safer environment not only for patients, but also for staff members and visitors.

The following is a summary of the highlights of each chapter:

- **Chapter 1: Elements of a Just Culture**—summarizes why the concept of a just culture came into being and explains the reasons behind reporting adverse events and the difference it has made to staff members and patients

- **Chapter 2: Assess Your Organization**—provides ideas and tools that can and should be used to help determine where an organization is in the just culture process and helps determine what still needs to be done

- **Chapter 3: Planning the Change**—identifies what actions and personnel specifically are needed in order to effect organizational change

- **Chapter 4: Just Culture Concepts: Reporting, QI, and Transparency**—discusses in detail what a just culture looks like, including how reporting can be effective, how quality improvement efforts can improve, and what part transparency plays in a just and safe culture

- **Chapter 5: Implementation Strategies**—offers ideas and recommendations for successful strategies used to implement a just culture approach

- **Chapter 6: Evaluating Change**—describes how to monitor and measure the effectiveness of the just culture concept

- **Chapter 7: Case Scenarios**—provides an example of an effective reporting process, a look at one hospital's efforts to reinvigorate its just culture efforts, and a touching personal story of a medication error

- **Chapter 8: Disclosure**—offers a discussion of "doing the right thing" in regard to the disclosure of adverse events

- **Appendix A: Nursing's Involvement in a Culture of Safety**—offers an in-depth literature-based resource for nursing's role in a culture of safety, including an expansive bibliography of resources

- **'Safe from Falls' Initiative Process and Outcomes Data Sample**—shows the actual data of one health system participating in the Maryland Patient Safety Center's "Safe from Falls" initiative. This is bonus material available at *www.hcpro.com/downloads/8752.*

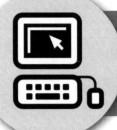

DOWNLOAD YOUR MATERIALS NOW

Readers of *Creating a Just Culture: A Nurse Leader's Guide* can download the figures included in this book by visiting the HCPro Web address below. At this link, you will find the following:

- Figure 1.1: States with adverse-event reporting systems

- Figure 2.1: Hospital survey on patient safety culture

- Figure 3.1: Dana-Farber Cancer Institute principles of a fair and just culture

- Figure 3.2: Incident reporting administrative policy

- Figure 3.3: Checklist for reviewing policies

- Figure 3.4: Staff education steps and checklist

- Figure 5.1: Just culture implementation timeline sample

- Figure 5.2: Three types of behavior

- Figure 6.1: Measuring progress with patient safety culture instruments

- Table 1: Domains of knowledge and skill sets to facilitate transformation to a culture of safety

- Table 2: Safety culture assessment survey tools

- 'Safe from Falls' Initiative Process and Outcomes Data Sample

We hope you will find the downloads useful.

www.hcpro.com/downloads/8752

Thank you for purchasing this product!

HCPro

1

Elements of a Just Culture

The concept of a "just culture" is not a new one, nor did it originate in the healthcare setting. The idea comes from the aviation industry and specifically from United Airlines. Crew resource management (CRM), which is a procedural system used when human error can have devastating effects, was first used to describe programs expressly designed to emphasize the need to change and correct deficiencies in cockpit crew behavior, specifically when it came to lack of assertiveness by junior crew members and the authoritarian behavior by captains. In fact, the National Transportation Safety Board had distinctly singled out the captain's failure to accept input from junior crew members and a lack of assertiveness by the flight engineer as causal factors in a United Airlines crash in 1978.

The CRM theory continues to be used in the aviation industry today, and more than 30 years later, the concept of this type of collaboration has finally trickled over into the medical community, largely due to folks such as John Nance, whose book about safety in human systems, *Blind Trust,*[1] is widely credited with helping to spark not only the universal acceptance of CRM principles in aviation, but also the earliest infusion of culture-changing lessons derived from aviation into medical practice. *Blind Trust* was instrumental in bringing to light for the American public some serious public issues in aviation safety. *Why Hospitals Should Fly: The Ultimate Flight Plan to Patient Safety and Quality Care,*[2] also authored by Nance, follows in that tradition. It discusses how these principles can be applied in the practice of medicine. CRM has evolved into what the medical community would now consider to be a just culture model, which has been expanded on by David Marx, an engineer and attorney who began his career as a Boeing aircraft design engineer. While at Boeing, Marx organized a human factors and safety group that proved to be quite successful. In 1997, he started a research and consulting practice focusing on the management of human error through the integration of systems engineering, human factors, and the law, otherwise known today as what he terms "a just culture."

These ideas have begun to infiltrate the healthcare field in new and exciting ways. A just culture can help your organization toward safer and better quality care, with a high potential of also creating a more satisfying place to work.

National Emphasis on Patient Safety

Ever since the Institute of Medicine (IOM) published *To Err is Human: Building a Safer Health System* in November 1999, there has been an ever-increasing focus on patient safety in the United States. According to the report, at least "44,000–98,000 people die in hospitals each year as a result of medical errors that could have been prevented."[3] To that end, a movement to improve patient safety across the country was initiated, particularly in light of several very publicized cases—the first being a medication error, specifically a massive overdose of a powerful anticancer drug that resulted in the death of 39-year-old Betsy Lehman in March 1995. The second was the amputation of the wrong leg of 51-year-old Willie King and the third was the death of 8-year-old Ben Kolb in December 1995 following a medication error that occurred during what should have been a relatively simple outpatient procedure. The fourth was that of miscommunication, resulting in the administration of three times the appropriate dosage of methadone that resulted in the death of 18-month-old Josie King in January 2001.

These events ultimately led to the passage of the Patient Safety and Quality Improvement Act of 2005. This act created patient safety organizations that collect, aggregate, and analyze event data that are reported voluntarily and confidentially in an effort to identify possible patterns and trends, which can then be used to develop and implement measures to prevent patient harm and promote patient safety without fear of reprisals.

With patient safety in the national spotlight, healthcare organizations have been forced to look at current practices and processes that may have facilitated the occurrence of an error rather than at the individuals who actually committed the error. Usually, nine times out of 10, the error was more process-related than people-related. Consequently, over the past 10 years there has been a growing trend toward creating leadership tracks in patient safety practices at conferences and seminars for healthcare professionals.

Reporting Errors for a Just Culture

Lucien Leape, MD, Harvard School of Public Health professor and patient safety expert, said in testimony before Congress on the Healthcare Research and Quality Act of 1999 that the "greatest impediment to error prevention is that we punish people for making mistakes." This is substantiated in the article entitled "The Perceptions of Just Culture Across Disciplines in Healthcare," which showed that when surveyed, at least 50% of the respondents acknowledge that when an incident occurs, someone will be blamed first, before an investigation has actually determined how and why the event occurred.[4]

And, if the medical community honestly acknowledged it, Leape's comments would, at least from the average community hospital nurse's perspective, definitely held true up until the past five to 10 years. Punishing people for making mistakes discourages them from reporting errors, preventing further error prevention.

The IOM report suggested the implementation of a two-tiered event reporting system: the mandatory approach, which requires state governments to oversee the collection of data pertaining to those adverse events that resulted in, or contributed to, the serious injury, illness, or death of a patient who was admitted to a hospital; and the voluntary approach, which focuses more on those repetitive errors that occur much more often but usually result in minimal or no harm and usually occur as a result of a flawed systems process.

Additionally, to encourage more robust reporting of these types of events and to reassure reporters that the information contained in the report would not be used against them in a medical malpractice liability claim or disciplinary proceeding, the federal Agency for Healthcare Research and Quality (AHRQ) included provisions in the Patient Safety Act for ensuring the maintenance of the data's confidentiality, as well as the data's protection from discovery with respect to any information reported, both of which were included in the final congressional act that was passed.

History of reporting

Reporting an adverse event, or "incident reporting," was originally initiated by the medical malpractice insurance industry in the 1970s in response to the medical malpractice crisis at the time when, generally speaking, payouts to claimants exceeded premiums and hospitals were either closing or being bought out by conglomerates like HCA Healthcare and Tenet Healthcare Corporation and physicians were exiting their practices in droves because they could no longer afford to pay their premiums. The industry created the written reporting mechanism as a way for healthcare providers to notify the insurance company whenever they thought that what is known as a "potentially compensable event" occurred. This type of event could very well lead to a malpractice claim or lawsuit.

Reporting such events allowed the company to set a reserve, where a certain amount of money was set aside for possible settlement of a claim—the specific amount determined by the type of injury, sympathy factor of the claimant, what associated medical expenses could be expected and how much they would cost, the value of lost wages, and other factors. At that time, hospital risk management departments were established, more or less, to reactively manage claims that were already made or would most likely potentially be made against the hospital, and employees were encouraged to report events that could lead to claims or lawsuits.

Employees were not necessarily encouraged to proactively report those errors that occurred repetitively, as these were considered to be careless in nature and identifying them was construed as punitive. Additionally, if an employee actually did complete an incident report to let risk

 Creating a Just Culture

management know of a potentially compensable event, or that the possibility that a lawsuit or claim might be filed, there was minimal, if any, effort to determine whether there was a system or process problem. It was just assumed that the individual involved was careless or not paying attention, and the action taken to address the issue at hand was usually to counsel, suspend, or even terminate the employee. This process did not allow for an evaluation of the event to determine whether there was actually a process problem versus a people problem, nor did it offer a mechanism by which a process improvement activity could be initiated once a cause was determined. There was no opportunity for the development of steps or an action plan that could be taken to ensure that there would not be a recurrence of such an event in the future.

State reporting

From an individual hospital's perspective, incident reporting is a critical component of any risk management program because it helps risk managers to be cognizant of unsafe systems that may need to be addressed, to analyze data and report findings of possible patterns and trends, and to track any actions taken to improve care once a problem has been identified. From a risk prevention perspective, this system is also used to report near misses—those events that could have reached the patient—not just those events that actually did reach the patient (whether or not there was harm). Reporting of these events allows risk management to investigate these types of events more closely to determine whether there are system breakdowns that contribute to their repetitive occurrence and address them before harm actually befalls a patient.

From a public reporting perspective, there are currently 26 states that have adverse-event reporting requirements, most of which require reporting of serious, most often preventable ,events that if made public would cause great concern to the community. Most states requiring the reporting of these types of events refer to the National Quality Forum's list of serious adverse events, which can be found online *(www.qualityforum.org/projects/completed/sre/fact-sheet.asp)*. There is no federal requirement for reporting. Each state that does require reporting has its own hospital-specific definitions of just what should be reported as serious events, which ultimately does not allow for even the most rudimentary aggregation of valid data. However, all states do have one thing in common: At the individual organizational level as well as at the state level, the organizations and the state authorities evaluate and analyze their own adverse-event data, identify the major areas of concern that need further investigation and analysis, and then work toward the design and implementation of new and improved processes, all in an effort to promote patient safety and prevent patient harm.

See Figure 1.1 for a list of states with hospital adverse-event reporting requirements, including what is required to be reported.

FIGURE
1.1

States with adverse-event reporting systems

State	Year System Began	Reportable Event List	Agency Receiving Reports	Number of Adverse Events Reported in 2006
California	2007	Modified NQF*	Department of Public Health, Office of Licensing and Certification	N/A
Colorado	1988	State determined	Department of Public Health and Environment, Health Facilities and Emergency Medical Services Division	391
Connecticut	2002	Modified NQF	Department of Public Health	240
District of Columbia	2007	Modified NQF	Health Regulation and Licensing Administration	N/A
Florida	1998	State determined	Agency for Healthcare Administration, Florida Center for Policy Analysis	716
Georgia	2003	State determined	Department of Human Resources, Office of Regulatory Services	136
Indiana	2006	NQF	Department of Health	79
Kansas	1988	State determined	Department of Health and Environment	22
Maine	2004	State determined	Department of Health and Human Services, Division of Licensing and Regulatory Services	24
Maryland	2004	State determined	Department of Health and Mental Hygiene, Office of Health Care Quality	174
Massachusetts	1980	State determined	Department of Public Health, Division of Health Care Quality	782
Minnesota	2003	NQF	Department of Health	140
Nevada	2005	State determined	State Health Division, Bureau of Health Planning and Statistics	188
New Jersey	2005	Modified NQF	Department of Health and Senior Services	450
New York	1985	State determined	Department of Health, Office of Health Systems Management	16,442
Ohio	2007	State determined	Department of Health, Office of Health Systems Management	N/A
Oregon	2006	Modified NQF	Patient Safety Commission	N/A a
Pennsylvania	2004	State determined	Patient Safety Authority	6,232 b
Rhode Island	1994	State determined	Department of Health, Division of Environmental and Health Services Regulation, Office of Facilities Regulation	271
South Carolina	1976	State determined	Department of Health and Environmental Control	N/A
South Dakota	1987	State determined	Department of Health	6
Tennessee	2000	State determined	Department of Health, Division of Healthcare Facilities	3,585
Utah	2001	Modified NQF	Department of Health	N/A
Vermont	2007	NQF	Department of Health	N/A
Washington	2006	Modified NQF	Department of Health	N/A a
Wyoming	2005	Modified NQF	Department of Health, Preventive Health and Safety Division	13

Source: Office of Inspector General analysis of States' legislation, statutes and regulations, forms, and 26 interviews, 2008.

* NQF is the National Quality Forum List of Serious Reportable Events.

a = States began collecting data in mid-2006 and, therefore, could not report complete data for the year.

b = This range does not include the number of near misses reported to Pennsylvania in 2006.

N/A = Not available; States did not provide the number of adverse event reports for 2006.

For example, in March 2004, Maryland mandated that every hospital had to have a formal patient safety program in place with a designated patient safety officer and required that all level 1 events be reported to the Department of Health and Mental Hygiene's Office of Healthcare Quality. Level 1 events are defined as those serious injuries, illnesses, or deaths either contributed by or resulting from the actions of hospital representatives, as determined by the organization, or conditions lasting longer than seven days and/or conditions that are still present at the time of discharge. Examples of the types of level 1 events are as follows:

- Death or serious disability related to the use of anticoagulants

- Death or serious disability related to the failure to maintain a patient's airway

- Death or serious disability as result of an unanticipated complication

- Death or serious disability related to a delay in treatment

- Unanticipated fetal or neonatal death or disability

- Misdiagnosis

The law also requires that a root cause analysis (RCA) of these events be conducted and an action plan be developed and submitted for evaluation and approval within 60 days of the date of the report.

Challenges to reporting

Suzanne C. Beyea notes in an article published in the April 2002 issue of *AORN Journal*, entitled "Reporting Medical Errors and Adverse Events," that the two main reasons errors are not reported as they should be are fear and a lack of belief that reporting can actually lead to improvements in the quality of patient care provided.[5] In fact, in one 2004 Institute of Safe Medication Practices survey conducted at the University of Alberta Hospital in Canada, when staff members were questioned about why they were uncomfortable with completing incident reports, "they readily admitted their reluctance to submit incident reports, citing concerns that they would be judged to be an inadequate practitioner and/or held responsible for the incident."[6]

In the past, healthcare workers have often been afraid that if they complete the report, they will face disciplinary action because, historically, patients generally believe that healthcare providers do not make mistakes. Many leaders in organizations believe in a culture of perfectionism and most providers feel enormous pressure to be right all of the time, with no exceptions, despite the fact that providers are human and will, at least one time in their careers, commit an error. When they do commit an error, most providers will spend a great deal of time feeling tremendous guilt and shame, failing to accept that there were system failures that allowed the provider to commit the error in the first place. Not to mention that if an error resulted in moderate-to-significant patient harm, there is the additional worry that a lawsuit will follow.

Many fear that whatever is documented in the incident report will be made available to the plaintiff's counsel and divulged in open court, leaving providers to believe their reputation is at stake. Additionally, if there is a payment made to the plaintiff, the provider will have to be reported to the National Practitioner Data Bank, creating an increase in medical malpractice insurance premium. In many cases, providers often end up either limiting privileges to lower-risk specialties or not performing potentially high-risk procedures—that is, if they stay in medicine at all.

This type of culture—in which medical professionals are viewed as infallible—is slowly but surely changing. The healthcare field is beginning to allow the reporting of events without reprisals while still holding persons accountable for what is determined as at-risk behavior. However, as much as healthcare organizations may want to change practices in order to more accurately reflect these current standards of care, providers are finding out that changing behavior and practice in order to improve the quality of care provided is a painstakingly hard road to follow. Data needs to be displayed, and information regarding any necessary follow-up actions must be communicated back to the provider. Additionally, actual improvements need to be seen in the provision of care or staff will often wonder why they bothered to report an event in the first place.

Case study: The effect of public reporting

Each of the past five years in Maryland reflects an increase in the number of events reported, which, according to the Office of Healthcare Quality (OHCQ), "does not necessarily mean that errors are occurring more frequently but may represent greater compliance on behalf of the hospitals and a

Creating a Just Culture

continued collaboration between OHCQ and Maryland hospitals, thereby increasing the reporting of events."[7] And, despite initial reticence on the part of the hospitals to share sentinel event information, over the years, Maryland hospitals have actually affirmed the need to critically analyze the cause(s) behind the errors, as this has definitely enabled them to more objectively evaluate and, if necessary, revise their systems and processes to ensure that proper checks and balances are in place to avoid mistakes reaching the patient.

These regulations have also resulted in hospital leadership taking a more "active role in reviewing the RCA submitted by their facilities in response to a Level 1 adverse event,"[8] and, as such, hospital leaders have now accepted the ultimate responsibility for ensuring that a change in culture must take place so that better quality care is provided to their community's patients. Senior leadership also acknowledges that:

> *Open communication among hospital disciplines and with the affected patient and family is key to a successful patient safety program. The inability or reluctance to disclose events is one of the most common root causes that can lead to system failures. Including the patient and the family in the RCA process can also be valuable in improving processes and future patient outcomes.*[9]

Additionally, the data collected by the OHCQ has provided some valuable information in regard to the types of events that are occurring across the state.

Maryland's Patient Safety Center follows how the AHRQ recommends state patient safety programs are to be structured. As discussed previously, the OHCQ requires mandatory reporting of specific events, while the Maryland Patient Safety Center (MPSC) focuses more on what is voluntarily reported. To that end, an electronic adverse-event reporting system was developed and offered to all Maryland hospitals, of which six have chosen to voluntarily report all events (actual, as well as near misses or good catches) that had the potential to cause a significant adverse outcome because of a process or system failure, but did not either through intervention or, in many cases, pure luck. These data are collected through the MPSC and aggregately reported at its annual patient safety conference, held every spring in Baltimore. This information helps the MPSC to identify patterns and trends regarding the types of errors occurring in what may be a statistically valid representation of all Maryland hospitals, which is then presented at the conference. The information can then be utilized in institutions across the state to assist with developing better processes that will proactively and simultaneously prevent the error from occurring and promote patient safety.

When we first started collecting data back in July 2006, we identified that medication errors were the most reported type of event, followed by falls. It was also reported that 97% of medication errors resulted in no patient harm. However, we did find that in about 20% of falls reported, patient harm was noted. Injuries could have been as minor as an abrasion or as serious as a resulting subdural hematoma, but if there was documentation of a patient sustaining any type of injury, it was considered to be patient harm. Because there were only about 850 events reported, no other analysis or conclusions could be made.

In 2008, the 2007 aggregate data was presented at the annual patient safety conference and, again, the same findings were identified, only now there were more than 4,000 records. This time, it was noted that about 24% of patients who fell sustained an injury of some sort. That being said, just a short time later, we began to look specifically at the falls data to determine what other activities or opportunities we could explore at the state level that we could share with our member hospitals in an effort to reduce both the frequency as well as the severity of patient injuries.

One of the first things we did was to share the data with the OHCQ to determine whether there may be a correlation between Level 1 event data and the MPSC's voluntary reporting data, which proved to be extremely useful in the development of the state's "Safe from Falls" initiative. "Safe from Falls" is a statewide project introduced in September 2009 to address the increasingly alarming reports related to patient falls—both Level 1 events and those reported as near misses. The initiative includes data collection from the implementation of process measures. By healthcare entities putting into place consistent and standardized policies, procedures, and protocols, the hope is that reported outcomes, not only from hospitals but from long-term care and home care entities as well, will show improvement.

Although it is too soon to know whether this initiative has definitively had a positive effect on frequency and/or severity of the events reported, the awareness of the initiative itself, and the ability of the facilities to be able to collaborate with each other, share their best practices, and compare themselves with similar facilities, has definitely shown that there is a shared culture of patient safety among all the participants, at least with respect to patient falls, and that makes for a huge win-win all across Maryland. A sample of reports provided to all MSPC falls initiative participants, which allow hospitals to see how they are progressing both individually as well as compared to the other participants, with respect to both outcomes and process measures, can be found in the 'Safe from Falls' Initiative Process and Outcomes Data Sample bonus material available at *www.hcpro.com/ downloads/8752.*

It is important to note that in reviewing the incident data reported after the falls initiative was introduced, the amount of laboratory errors has seesawed back and forth, with falls for the second type of event most often reported. A similar finding has been reported by the Pennsylvania Patient Safety Authority, and that organization is looking more closely at the data to see if further action is warranted at the statewide level; it may be time for the MPSC to take similar action.

Defining Your Current Culture

Other recommendations made in the IOM report include defining, as well as raising, the performance standards for healthcare patient safety professionals and encouraging health insurance purchasers and insurers to set minimum safety requirements when making their contracting decisions, which in essence provides monetary incentives for the performance of safe, quality patient care.

The one recommendation in healthcare that has proved to be the most challenging for hospitals is that they must develop a "culture of safety" within their own entity, meaning they need to focus more on the concept of workforce performance improvement, specifically ensuring that the organization has made patient safety a strategic priority, a message that absolutely needs to be driven home over and over again from the top down—from board members to senior leadership to the medical staff to directors to supervisors to managers and, most importantly, to the frontline staff—because if they see that the commitment is there from the top down, there is more unity and buy-in for the concept. If managers do not tout the message, the message tends to lose importance.

However, before an organization can even begin to develop a culture of safety, it needs to determine just what the current organizational culture is, and that involves evaluating factors such as the current state of beliefs, values, and attitudes that are shared by a group. In other words, the foundation of the culture within the organization, be it positive or negative, most assuredly acts as a guide as to how employees will behave in the workplace. Simply put, it is how things actually are done versus how things *should* be done.

Additionally, an organization needs to consider the culture of its individual employees as well as that of each department or clinical service. Obviously, behavior is influenced or determined by what actions are rewarded and acceptable within the workplace and what actions or behaviors are not. For example, if a pharmacist makes a dispensing error, and that error is caught as a near miss by another pharmacist, and the correct medication is then sent to the floor with no one the wiser, chances are it won't ever be reported as an incident. The belief is that this was not an error because it was caught before it got the to floor or to the patient. But a critical factor is ignored here: An error did occur and there should be questions asked about the error. Why did the error occur in the first place? Was this a one-time error or has it occurred with some frequency? Staff need to understand that the potential for patient harm is still present, because the same error might occur again due to a potential system error. There needs to be a willingness on the part of the pharmacy department to commit to changing their attitude and to acknowledge that an error occurred and that it needs to be reported so current processes can be evaluated.

By determining what the current culture is, the organization can begin to address how attitudes and behaviors can be changed and how the culture can be transitioned to one that is more patient safety focused. Keep in mind that an organization's transition to a more patient-safety-conscious culture will need to proceed by steps and this process will take time.

This process is described by R. Westrum in his article "A Typology of Organizational Cultures," published in *Quality & Safety in Health Care* in December 2004.[10] He describes the three phases as being pathological, bureaucratic, and generative. Pathological is when an organization is secretive and unwilling to share information, refuses to consider new ideas or concepts, and covers up any adverse outcomes or negative behaviors. The next phase is bureaucratic in nature. This is when an organization's leaders "talk the talk" but don't "walk the walk." The organization may say it has a just and patient-safety-focused culture, but in reality it merely tolerates when new ideas are brought

 Creating a Just Culture

to the table; it will not act on them. In fact, this organization usually ignores the information provided in the first place. Eventually the organization gets to the next phase, known as the generative or learning phase. This is where the organization is always looking for information that will help them become a safer place for their employees, patients, and visitors. New ideas are welcomed and failures are evaluated for systemic issues, not just blamed on the employee involved in the event.

Leadership plays a critical role in making the case for patient safety, because without its support of the concepts and actions taken to promote patient safety and prevent patient harm throughout the organization, efforts will all be in vain and the program will be destined to fail. However, by establishing a culture that supports and advances patient safety and, more specifically, supports the discussion of errors so that lessons can be learned from them, the organization is supporting a just culture approach. This approach encourages a multidisciplinary communication process and a nonpunitive approach to event reporting.

A just culture also holds managers and staff members accountable and responsible for establishing reliable improvements to processes of care and adhering to them. In his book *Managing the Risks of Organizational Accidents*, James Reason says that a true culture of safety is, in fact, made up of several cultures that are just and fair—they report, learn, inform, and are flexible. According to Reason, a just culture is one in which the atmosphere is one of trust and it encourages and rewards staff members for providing essential safety-related information but, more importantly, is also very clear about what is acceptable and unacceptable behavior.[11]

David Marx says that errors occur because people exhibit one of the three following behaviors:

1. An inadvertent action of doing other than what should have been done, such as a slip or a mistake.

2. At-risk behavior, or an action that increases risk where either the risk isn't recognized or is believed to be justified, even when it is known to be the wrong action to take.

3. Reckless behavior, when the individual consciously chooses to disregard a substantial and unjustifiable risk. It is this behavior that is managed via remedial or disciplinary action, not the previous two behaviors.[12]

Once these behaviors are understood, there should be an ethical imperative for reporting adverse events to ensure that the management of the event occurred according to established protocols, to notify the proper personnel, to investigate why the event happened, to study the possible causes and contributing factors, and to design and implement better processes that will prevent the occurrence of similar events. Why? Because it is the right thing to do and we as healthcare professionals have a responsibility to our patients to keep them safe while they are under our care.

Recruitment and Staff Retention

One of the benefits of improving the quality of patient care is improved employee turnover rates. At Hackensack (NJ) University Medical Center, an excellent practice environment has resulted in a nurse employee turnover rate of 6.3%, below the national average, saving the hospital approximately $45,000–$68,000 in recruitment and training expenses for each nurse. There appears to be a direct correlation between the organization's turnover rate and its adoption of a culture that supports patient safety.[13]

It is widely known that healthcare professionals face a variety of work-related hazards during the course of their day, so it is no wonder they sustain musculoskeletal injuries, infections, and mental stress, just to name a few work-related occupational conditions. Healthcare workers also experience more stress and fatigue than many other occupations. They may feel overworked, with an ever increasing workload, and at times, they may work in what seem to them as unsafe conditions. When healthcare workers feel their environment is not conducive to being able to provide safe, high-quality care to their patients, they are usually unhappy. It becomes clear that employee well-being and how employees feel about their environment has a direct impact on patient safety. You see, it seems that if an employee works in an environment that does not promote patient safety, does not support just culture initiatives, does not address inadequate staffing, and does not promote effective communication, the more likely it is that the employee will commit an error, because systems failures are not evaluated. In other words, if an employee doesn't feel that the organization supports him or her in his or her efforts to do a good job, then why should the employee support the organization? Additionally, if the organization doesn't support patient safety initiatives, there is a good chance the employee will not stay long and will move to an environment more conducive to promoting patient safety and preventing patient harm.

To counter the previous discussion, it seems that low employee turnover rates appear to be directly related to "lower failure-to-rescue rates, lower inpatient mortality rates, shorter hospital stays, and fewer work-related injuries."[14] A happier, healthier workplace results in less stress to the employee, thereby eliminating those aspects of the workplace considered to be "toxic." So, what is considered to be a toxic work environment? In truth, any work environment can become toxic if, it includes, or even promotes, behavior that negatively affects others in the same workplace.

Not only that, but if this type of behavior occurs on a fairly routine basis, and is not addressed promptly and appropriately by the organization's leadership, it can affect far more than just employee retention—it can also affect how coworkers handle certain stressful situations. Negative behavior can also affect the long-range plans and reputation of the entire organization. Additionally, it makes it difficult to build a culture of teamwork, particularly when the employee retention rate is directly related to pervasive adverse behavior.

Symptoms of a toxic work environment can include increased absenteeism, health problems and accidents, more resignations, and the loss of talented employees. Although in some cases the toxicity can be related to just one individual, in many cases systemic factors can reinforce toxic behavior or practices, particularly if senior management chooses to look the other way or exhibits indifference to the inappropriate actions. The good news is that, most of the time, once the behavior is made known to human resources, the environment is usually turned around fairly quickly, particularly when senior leadership is made aware of the costs to the organization if these situations are not addressed, which include lost productivity, higher-than-expected employee turnover, and, of course, the potential legal liability.

On the other hand, when an employee feels that he or she works in a healthy work environment where the organization values both patient and employee safety, the employee is more likely to provide high-quality patient care. The bottom line is that supporting a positive workplace also supports quality patient care. To that end, we should do everything we can to make the work environment of our staff as welcoming and inviting as possible. The rewards will be beyond expectations, because when organizations have a reputation for "playing nice in the sandbox," relationships are established that, in most cases, will lead to better opportunities and almost always lead to improved patient care.

Staff and Patient Education

Lastly, the organization should educate patients about their own roles in protecting themselves from medical errors. By knowing about their illness or condition, which medications they are taking and what they look like, and reminding hospital personnel and the medical staff to wash their hands before and after the physical examination or assessment, patients are playing a part in ensuring a culture of safety throughout the organization, not to mention the direct impact in their own safety while in the care of others. This open communication between staff members and patients can make the difference between a positive outcome or an adverse event. In fact, staff should consider inviting patients and their families to speak directly to nursing about any perceptions they may have about the safety of their own care and to be willing to share experiences if, in fact, a medical error has occurred to them or to a loved one at some time in the past.

In fact, communication breakdowns between care providers themselves as well as between care providers and patients can, and often do, put patient safety at great risk when concerns about the safety of the care being provided are not made known clearly. Additionally, by empowering staff members with a clear understanding of their role in the promotion of patient safety, they will feel that they actually do make a difference in ensuring that patients are safe while in their care, their motivation to go beyond the call of their own professional duty increases, and they are encouraged to take responsibility for their own actions.

From the patients' perspective, by being actively engaged in patient safety efforts, they can and should be able to initiate conversations with their healthcare providers regarding simple things, such as asking the reason why a certain medication has been ordered for them or asking the provider to wash his or her hands before any examination.

Families should also be able to utilize communication efforts, such as calling a rapid response team whenever they suspect the patient's condition has changed or asking for instructions on how to take care of a patient's needs once he or she discharged. In 2007, The Joint Commission included in their scoring standards a requirement strongly encouraging interdisciplinary communication and collaboration that includes patients and their families, so that they are actively involved in their own care as a patient safety strategy, known as their Speak Up™ campaign. (Information about this initiative can be found at *www.jointcommission.org/PatientSafety/SpeakUp.*) Additionally, the AHRQ has developed a program known as "Questions Are the Answer," along with a fact sheet entitled *20 Tips to Help Prevent Medical Errors.* This four-page document (found at *www.ahrq.gov/consumer/20tips.htm*) is a helpful guide that can be referenced by patients and families. Preliminary studies seem to indicate that when patients take a more participative role in their care, their own safety seems to improve. Furthermore, when patients and staff are effectively and comfortably communicating about the care being provided, and staff is more confident about being able to discuss areas of concern without fear of being chastised, the more an organization demonstrates that it has embraced a just culture approach.

The First Steps of Your Journey

It is important for hospitals and staff members to be continuously reminded that the primary strategic focus for any healthcare entity should be patient-centered care that keeps patients safe. Patient-centered care should include a mechanism whereby hospital personnel and/or the medical staff are comfortable reporting any medical error through the appropriate channels in a continuous effort to improve the quality of care provided. It is also imperative that staff members be involved in the initiative for organizational cultural change, because if the staff isn't on board with the concept—even if the governing body and senior leadership are—the initiative will fail.

Now that the need for change is recognized, it is time to get started. This handbook will guide the way with a hands-on approach, providing information, techniques, and tools to assist organizations as they move through the process of culture change. This is an exciting journey, although at times it can be quite challenging. Still, staff members want to do the right things for their patients; they want to provide the right care to the right patient at the right time and in the right setting. We expect that this handbook will help to do just that, particularly with respect to those responsible for direct, hands-on patient care. The overall goal of a just culture is to look beyond the individual when an error occurs. Making the individual aware of outcomes and holding the individual responsible for learning from his or her mistakes and to performing according to preset expectations in the future, while at the same time evaluating the processes leading up to the error, identifying breaks in those processes, and correcting them, the organization demonstrates its commitment to objectively understanding why the error occurred and to adopting a systematic approach for addressing errors without staff fearing there will be adverse consequences to them, personally or professionally.

Your action plan for getting started should include:

- Assessing your organization's current culture of patient safety via a survey of a patient safety culture.

- Once findings are received, developing a plan for addressing those areas identified as needing improvement.

- Once the plan has been implemented, communicating to staff just what the plan is, what is required of them to ensure its success, and publicizing efforts made throughout the organization.

- If policies, procedures, or protocols require revision, including staff in the revision process to ensure that practice reasonably adheres to policy.

- Communicating to and educating every staff member about all efforts currently being made to transition to a more just and patient-focused culture, including any changes in policy, expected performance, and behavior. A regular report on progress should be made to convey this throughout the organization. Encourage staff to ask questions about any specific areas of concern.

References

1. Nance, John. *Blind Trust.* William Morrow & Co., 1987.

2. Nance, John. *Why Hospitals Should Fly: The Ultimate Flight Plan to Patient Safety and Quality Care.* Second River Healthcare Press, 2008.

3. Kohn, Linda T., Corrigan, Janet M., and Donaldson, Molla S. *To Err Is Human: Building a Safer Health System, an Executive Summary.* National Academy of Sciences, Committee on Quality of Health Care in America, Institute of Medicine, p. 1.

4. von Thaden, Terry, etc. "The Perception of Just Culture Across the Disciplines in Healthcare." *Human Factors and Ergonomics Society Annual Meeting Proceedings,* Human Factors and Ergonomics Society, 2006. pp. 964–968(5)

5. Beyea, Suzanne. "Reporting medical errors and adverse events – research corner," *AORN Journal,* April (2002): 1.

6. Zboril-Benson, Leone, and Magee, Bernice. "How quality improvement projects influence organizational culture." *Healthcare Quarterly* 8, October Special Issue (2005): 1.

7. Office of Healthcare Quality, Department of Health and Mental Hygiene. *Maryland Hospital Patient Safety Program Annual Report Fiscal Year 2009,* 2009.

8. Ibid.

9. Ibid.

10. Westrum, R. "A typology of organizational cultures." *Quality & Safety in Health Care,* December (2004).

11. Reason, James. *Managing the Risks of Organizational Accidents.* Ashgate Publishing, 1997.

12. Marx, David. *Whack-a-Mole: The Price We Pay for Expecting Perfection.* By Your Side Studios, 2009.

13. Yassi, Annalee and Hancock, Tina. "Patient safety – worker safety: Building a culture of safety to improve healthcare worker and patient well-being," *Healthcare Quarterly* 8, October Special Issue (2005): 33.

14. Ibid.

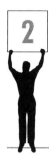

Assess Your Organization

LEARNING OBJECTIVES

- Define culture

- Identify ways to assess organizational culture

Assessing your organization to find out where you stand as a culture is critical to understanding your next steps on your journey toward a just culture. Understanding what culture is can help you understand what your organization's culture is like.

What Is Culture?

How would you define *culture*? If you asked two people who lived in the same town, you would most likely get two different answers, depending on family history; the country, state, or province in which each was born; race; gender; where each person went to school; what his or her parents did for a living; and many other factors. Culture tells us how we should behave, dress, talk, and react to a certain set of circumstances as we grow and mature within our own community.

The Free Dictionary defines culture as "language, values, customs, and aesthetics of an individual or a group of people." Culture influences attitudes about health and healthcare. Culture is learned and noninstinctive; an individual can begin his or her life learning about one set of values and beliefs and, for whatever reason, this person could be placed into a completely new environment with a totally different culture and, in time, would learn to accept the new one as his or her own.

Cultures do not remain static. All cultures will change over time, but the rate of cultural change varies from society to society and environment to environment, even when these different environments are not that far apart geographically. Additionally, adopting new traits or abandoning old ones will have a direct impact on those remaining unchanged, because they have, up to this point, been interconnected—which is why there can be a significant resistance to change and why change can often be very difficult for individuals within the culture to accept. Why? Because we don't realize how much we are used to and fond of our own culture until faced with a change that is significantly alien or foreign to us and, as such, we may not believe that particular change was a good thing, particularly if it wasn't our own idea. When we are closed-minded about change, we tend to have a negative prejudice against it, and that prevents us from understanding or appreciating other cultures or societies. Furthermore, this prejudice prevents us from effectively communicating with others, leading to misunderstandings and mistrust between the involved parties.

What needs to be understood is that change isn't necessarily a bad thing, nor are the people advocating change necessarily bad people. In most instances, not all of the old culture should be eliminated, particularly with respect to certain traditions, as they help to keep the history of a particular culture alive and not forgotten, preserving certain customs for future generations to appreciate.

How Culture Affects Care

Each of us has grown into who we are today because of the culture in which we were raised. Healthcare providers have their own unique culture, one that is usually very different from that of their patients. Healthcare providers are socialized into the culture of their specific profession and work environment and, based on their specialized education, they have a particular way of viewing certain aspects of life that is very different from that of their patients. In fact, healthcare providers

 Creating a Just Culture

even speak a different language than their patients—one of medical jargon. Traditionally, we as patients have come to respect doctors to the extent that we are in awe of their status as experts who can guide us toward maintaining, as well as improving, our own health and well-being.

Furthermore, most patients look up to healthcare providers as being almost omnipotent since we do, for the most part, rely on them to properly diagnose and treat us without question, and without ever making a mistake. Right from the beginning, there are cultural gaps between providers and patients. Providers adhere quite strongly to the western system of healthcare delivery, which is predominantly based on science and, until recently, did not take much stock in eastern, nontraditional methods of providing care, which also consider taking care of the patient as a human being and tailoring care to meet the specific needs of the patient. To that end, providers face a tremendous amount of stress to meet our expectations, particularly when they are human and, as such, are bound to occasionally make a mistake. How they perceive their own culture has a large impact on how they communicate what happened when a mistake is actually made.

When a provider does make a mistake, and a patient is harmed, how this is managed can and does tell a great deal about the culture of the provider, the patient and/or family, as well as the community. For example consider the following scenario:

> *A patient undergoes a cardiac catheterization to rule out any coronary artery disease, and he or she goes to his or her local, rural community hospital and the procedure is planned as an outpatient procedure. The patient expects to be discharged home later the same day. During the course of the procedure, a mistake is made—an artery is accidentally nicked with the catheterization needle, and the patient begins to lose a lot of blood. Because the mistake isn't recognized in a timely fashion, it causes a drop in the patient's blood pressure, and the patient goes into cardiac arrest and dies.*

If the physician is very autocratic in the procedure room, creating an atmosphere in which staff are very nervous about working with the physician, everyone involved might play a part in hiding mistakes. The providers may never tell the patient's family what, if anything, went wrong. If they are forced to admit something went wrong, there could be a million excuses as to why the artery got punctured, such as because there was an equipment malfunction, the staff didn't communicate to the provider that the patient's condition was deteriorating, or the patient's own anatomy was unique and, as such, the event occurrence was unavoidable. These reasons might be given if the physician and/or staff are fearful that disclosing the true error will result in the patient's family behaving irrationally and perhaps threatening bodily harm. Or, the provider and/or the hospital staff fear they will be solely blamed for the error and that extenuating circumstances will be disregarded. They might fear that because of this mistake or error, everyone's reputation will suffer, particularly the individual provider's, which could result in his or her future patient load being affected. This of course could affect his or her income, as well as his or her way of life, not to mention what it will probably do to all of the parties' medical malpractice liability insurance premiums.

If the hospital leadership have developed a very traditional culture, they might want to distance the hospital from the provider, going so far as to use the defense that because the physician is not employed, but was a contracted individual, the hospital shouldn't be held in any way responsible for the acts of the physician. This notion will tend to let the physician hang out to dry, without evaluating the possible underlying causes that produced the set of error-prone circumstances in the first place.

These outcome examples do not exemplify a just culture. Nowhere does the hospital take the time to understand all possible causes of the error. This does not mean that those staff members involved should be let off the hook, but if they are not given a chance to provide all the information that might be useful and then the hospital is not given a chance to improve itself by focusing on all causes and determining future prevention methods.

If we want to change that culture-of-blame scenario, we must begin to look at other possible causes besides human factors alone. Then we will actually begin to steer away from a culture of blame to one more willing to look outside the box and examine just why the error occurred in the first place. The assurance of patient safety depends on a healthcare delivery system providing better-quality patient care. In order to accomplish this, the entire organization, from the board of directors to frontline staff members, must be committed to learning from errors and understanding why they occurred. They must put systems in place to prevent errors from happening again, ultimately resulting in improved patient care and related outcomes.

Now, this does not, nor should it, absolve the individual from accepting responsibility for the part he or she may have played in the error's occurrence. Obviously, although the conditions may have been ripe for the event to occur, the individual also made choices that contributed to the final outcome—choices that, had the individual acted differently, might have altered the ultimate outcome. However, in most cases, the act was clearly not an intentional one done to purposefully harm the patient; more likely, it occurred because a policy or protocol was not followed and the individual provider needs to be made aware of his or her responsibility, held accountable for his or her actions, and reminded about the need to follow protocols.

Shared accountability

The individual should not be punished for an unintentional act to the extent that the individual is afraid his or her job may be in jeopardy, or that he or she becomes afraid to report future adverse events. We just want to make sure the provider learns from his or her mistakes so that similar events can be prevented from happening in the future. Therefore, it must be acknowledged that there are multiple factors relating to the occurrence of an adverse outcome and there are almost always multiple parties for which responsibility and accountability can be fully shared. Board governance, administration, and providers need to forget about living in their own vacuum or in different silos and instead begin to create an all-encompassing healthcare world for themselves, their patients, and their community—a world that values patient safety both in concept and in action.

The provision of healthcare can be daunting, and all parties involved in its delivery need to acknowledge and accept that there are inherent risks to providing care. Healthcare is more than just a science; it is also an art. The prevalent culture of an organization has a definitive impact on whether its patients are safe. It is, therefore, absolutely essential that a culture of safety be cultivated and, if necessary, behaviors changed to ensure that the risks to patients, staff, and community are minimized. Developing team-building communication techniques and treating each member of the healthcare team as an equal, learning from mistakes made in the past, and allowing the reporting of events to be a learning opportunity for others to help prevent similar events from happening in the future are just some of the ways in which a culture of safety can, and most often is, highly successful in ensuring that the ultimate goal for any healthcare provider is to "first, do no harm."

What a just culture looks like

So, how does an organization begin to move toward embracing this totally different way of thinking? Let's go back to that example of the cardiac catheterization case, but suppose now that a similar set of circumstances occurred under a more just culture. When the artery was first punctured, no one identified the event until the patient's blood pressure dropped; however, in this example, the minute the mistake is identified, the nurse quickly communicates to the physician that the patient's condition was deteriorating. The physician and staff continue to communicate with each other about what needs to be done, but despite all efforts, the patient still dies. This time, the entire healthcare team alerts risk management of the event, a quick debriefing meeting takes place before staff talks to the family, and then the team comes out to the waiting area to tell the patient's family exactly what happened, answering questions without blaming others, but each accepting responsibility for their own part in the event and supporting each other during the discussion. The conversation ends with letting the family know that the organization will conduct a more complete evaluation of the sequence of events surrounding the incident and will provide regular updates to the family regarding findings learned up to that point. The team tells the family that they will make themselves available if there are any questions and assures the family that the entire team involved will work together to develop an action plan designed to prevent similar events from happening in the future.

Successful organizations that promote patient safety and always work toward preventing patient harm through positive and continuous learning have incorporated a culture that has found a balance between improving processes and systems and fairly and justly addressing individual provider performance—in other words, a just culture.

Undertaking a Cultural Assessment

The first step to moving toward a just culture is to determine what kind of culture currently exists within the organization. The Joint Commission's leadership standard LD.03.01.01 states that leaders create and maintain a culture of safety and quality throughout the hospital. Furthermore, LD.03.01.01's first element of performance requires that leaders regularly evaluate the culture of safety and quality using valid and reliable tools. The easiest way healthcare entities can accomplish this is by conducting an initial, in-depth survey of patient survey culture to determine what the organization's current culture is and then conducting regular follow-up surveys to evaluate progress.

Creating a Just Culture

By conducting a survey, the organization determines whether its values are in accordance with a just culture. If it values safety, effectiveness of care, equity in the provision of care to all patients, and protecting and respecting the dignity of all who walk through the hospital doors, then it would probably be fairly safe to say that the organization is on the right track. In most instances, you can tell whether an organization values a just culture just by looking at a few practices. For example, an organization that does the following has demonstrated a culture of safety:

- All job descriptions include being accountable for ensuring patient safety during the course of performing their duties

- Incident reporting is valued to assist the organization with identifying possible patterns and trends and is promoted by the implementation of a user-friendly system

- There is an attitude of teamwork and open communication in which all team members are treated as equal partners in proving patient care, and they continuously exhibit behavior that allows staff to be comfortable drawing attention to potential hazards with out fear of reprisals

- Staff and leadership consider promoting patient safety and preventing patient harm as a clear top priority

Regardless of the type of facility, whether acute, long-term care, or home healthcare, the next step is to find out what worker and management perceptions and opinions are in regard to patient safety. There are a variety of ways in which this can be accomplished. Interviews with staff members can be conducted or questionnaires can be disseminated to staff members. Conducting interviews and scheduling in-person focus group meetings with each department, or scheduling them based on time frames, are usually the best ways to get the most honest results, provided appropriate individuals facilitate the groups and reassure folks that responses are kept confidential. Participants should also be reassured that there will be absolutely no punitive actions taken for being honest. Phone interviews can also be an effective tool, where randomly selected staff members from each department are called and asked a series of questions about their perception of the organization's current culture of safety that are recorded by the caller/surveyor. If using a formally developed, written survey tool, staff can either complete a paper form or take the survey online. Staff then complete and return the survey to the originator with the gathering of data usually taking somewhere between 30–60 days, depending on how long the organization would like have the survey tool available for staff to complete.

An example of a standardized survey tool can be found by going to *www.ahrq.gov* and clicking "Quality and Patient Safety." Responses are then collated and tabulated, then forwarded on to a data analyst to evaluate the findings. The evaluation is then reported to leadership for further discussion and decision-making. The information collected will usually prove to be quite valuable, particularly because in most cases the perspective of each group is usually vastly different from the others and distinctly emphasizes the disconnect between the groups, usually with senior leadership thinking there is more of a positive culture of safety within the organization and staff members feeling there is more of a punitive response whenever there is a medical error or near miss reported.

The key to getting fairly accurate responses back for measurement is to ensure anonymity of the respondents and accept that, in many cases, responses are not going to be favorable and, in fact, might be a bit caustic at times—and that's okay. Negative responses can tell just as good a story as positive ones, so it is important not to discount them and to include all comments made when a report of the findings is generated. The report should then be shared with the key individuals responsible for facilitating a change in organizational culture, such as senior leadership and/or middle management, who should then work with key staff members who have a true passion for patient safety and would like to be part of the change process by developing and implementing an action plan that will move the organization toward establishing a just culture. These folks should be representative of the organization as a whole and should include staff from all levels—board members, senior leadership, directors, and managers—as well as staff members and frontline staff from clinical and nonclinical areas. Examples of questionnaires can be found at the following websites:

- *www.chpso.org/just/cultsurv.pdf*

- *www.ahrq.gov/qual/patientsafetyculture/hospscanform.pdf*

- *www.ahrq.gov/qual/patientsafetyculture/hospdim.htm*

An excerpt of a sample survey is shown in Figure 2.1. This survey can be downloaded in its entirety at *www.hcpro.com/downloads/8752.*

 Creating a Just Culture

FIGURE 2.1

Hospital survey on patient safety culture

Instructions

This survey asks for your opinions about patient safety issues, medical error, and event reporting in your hospital and will take about 10 to 15 minutes to complete.

If you do not wish to answer a question, or if a question does not apply to you, you may leave your answer blank.

- An **_"event"_** is defined as any type of error, mistake, incident, accident, or deviation, regardless of whether or not it results in patient harm.
- **_"Patient safety"_** is defined as the avoidance and prevention of patient injuries or adverse events resulting from the processes of health care delivery.

SECTION A: Your Work Area/Unit

In this survey, think of your "unit" as the work area, department, or clinical area of the hospital where you spend _most_ of your work time or provide _most_ of your clinical services.

What is your primary work area or unit in this hospital? Select ONE answer.

☐ a. Many different hospital units/No specific unit

☐ b. Medicine (non-surgical)   ☐ h. Psychiatry/mental health   ☐ n. Other, please specify:

☐ c. Surgery   ☐ i. Rehabilitation

☐ d. Obstetrics   ☐ j. Pharmacy

☐ e. Pediatrics   ☐ k. Laboratory

☐ f. Emergency department   ☐ l. Radiology

☐ g. Intensive care unit (any type)   ☐ m. Anesthesiology

Please indicate your agreement or disagreement with the following statements about your work area/unit.

Think about your hospital work area/unit...	Strongly Disagree ▼	Disagree ▼	Neither ▼	Agree ▼	Strongly Agree ▼
1. People support one another in this unit	☐1	☐2	☐3	☐4	☐5
2. We have enough staff to handle the workload	☐1	☐2	☐3	☐4	☐5
3. When a lot of work needs to be done quickly, we work together as a team to get the work done	☐1	☐2	☐3	☐4	☐5
4. In this unit, people treat each other with respect	☐1	☐2	☐3	☐4	☐5
5. Staff in this unit work longer hours than is best for patient care	☐1	☐2	☐3	☐4	☐5

Source: Hospital Survey on Patient Safety Culture. April 2010. Agency for Healthcare Research and Quality, Rockville, MD. www.ahrq.gov/qual/patientsafetyculture/hospsurvindex.htm.

This survey can be downloaded in its entirety at www.hcpro.com/downloads/8752.

Reviewing Policies and Procedures

Another way to evaluate the type of culture that currently exists in an organization is by reviewing current policies and procedures relating to at least the following topics:

- Adverse-event reporting

- Sentinel-event reporting

- Patient-complaint reporting

- Reporting of potentially compensable events

- Transparency and disclosure of adverse events

- Performance of root cause and failure modes effects analyses

- Patient rights and responsibilities

- Chain of command

- Human resources policies and procedures relating to employee discipline

- Medical staff bylaws, rules, and regulations relating to the physician disciplinary action process

- Quality management program and plan

- Patient safety program and plan

- Risk management program and plan

- Administrative policies and procedures relating to quality, risk, and patient safety management

- Compliance policies relating to the management of grievances made by staff and/or patients

- Compliance policies relating to waiving payments for serious adverse events

 Creating a Just Culture

Policies and procedures should provide clear and distinct instructions for management of situations, with expert resource materials to support and recommend a specific and appropriate course of action to be taken, particularly for the new employees or less-experienced staff.

General policy language regarding the purpose of the policy should be consistent throughout all of the organization's policies and should not be in conflict with other policies, particularly with respect to patient safety efforts, including the support of a just culture.

Policy language that supports a just culture approach should include something similar to the following:

> *The ABC Hospital Center supports the framework of a "just culture," which encourages learning, openness, and fairness; the designing of safe systems; and the fair management of individual behavioral choices. A "just" culture is one that provides a fair and productive alternative to the two extremes of punitive or blame-free cultures, and balances the need to have a nonpunitive learning environment with the need to hold persons accountable for their actions. However, the ABC Hospital Center also acknowledges and accepts that although individuals should not be held accountable for system failures over which they had no control, the organization will not tolerate conscious disregard of another individual's safety, gross misconduct, or negligence (such as substance abuse while on duty, attempting to falsify or destroy legal medical documents/information).*[1]

Sample policies and procedures relating to many of the above topics can be accessed at several websites, including the ECRI Institute's website at *www.ecri.org* and specifically located in their healthcare risk control manuals; in the American Society for Healthcare Risk Management's *Risk Management Handbook for Health Care Organizations*, available at the American Society for Healthcare Risk Management (*www.ashrm.org*); the Agency for Healthcare Research and Quality website (*www.ahrq.gov*); and the National Patient Safety Foundation's website at *www.npsf.org*.

If this language is not included in your policies and procedures, it is fairly safe to assume that the organization's current culture does not promote staff members feeling comfortable about reporting adverse events or an openness to learning from the errors once they've been made known. If this is the case, then it is time for the organization to reevaluate what its strategic goals and objectives should be, for without including quality improvement and patient safety strategies as one of the organization's top priorities, the organization will never move to the next level of providing high-quality care in as safe a manner as is humanly possible. Once these priorities are established, then it is time to revise and update these policies to reflect that the organization is now dedicated to changing its approach toward a more fair and just way of addressing the management of adverse-event reporting.

Staff Education and Perception

Once these policies have been revised per your organization's individual policy review and revision process, all staff members—including the board of directors, senior leadership, the medical staff, and all hospital personnel—must be educated regarding what these changes are, how these new policies will be implemented, how their effectiveness will be measured and evaluated, and how progress is to be continuously reported back to reassure staff members that their feedback is valued and taken seriously.

Additionally, it is imperative that all healthcare providers are comfortable and confident that the organization will do everything in its power to protect all quality improvement and patient safety information from discovery if attempts are made by the legal system, regulatory agencies, or any other formal entities to obtain it. In all fairness to staff members, if they don't feel comfortable that what they report and communicate will absolutely stay within the hospital's four walls, despite knowing that reporting events is the right thing to do, it will be much more difficult for them to feel comfortable reporting events, particularly those in which they may have been involved, no matter how just the organization's culture really is. To that end, staff can be reassured when several citations of specific protections afforded by statute are included in policy and/or procedure language, similar to what follows:

> *Per the Patient Safety and Quality Improvement Act of 2005, federal legal privilege and confidentiality protections to information that is assembled and reported by providers to a PSO or developed by a PSO ("patient safety work product") for the conduct of patient safety activities has been afforded to information gathered during the investigation and evaluation of this event/ situation/potential quality issue or area of concern. Per this Act, the use of this information in*

 Creating a Just Culture

criminal, civil, and administrative proceedings is significantly limited. The Act includes provisions for monetary penalties for violations of confidentiality or privilege protections.

Additionally, the Act specifies the role of PSOs and defines "patient safety work product" and "patient safety evaluation systems," which is to focus on how patient safety event information is collected, developed, analyzed, and maintained. In addition, the Act has specific requirements for PSOs, such as:

- *PSOs are required to work with more than one provider.*

- *Eligible organizations include public or private entities, profit or not-for-profit entities, provider entities, such as hospital chains, and other entities that establish special components.*

- *Ineligible organizations include insurance companies or their affiliates.[2]*

References

1. Frankeberger, Gail M., and Turner, Bonnie B. "Changing from within – A journey toward just culture." Carilion Clinic, *www.vhqc.org/files/091029AJustCulture.pdf*.

2. The Patient Safety and Quality Improvement Act of 2005. Overview, June 2008. Agency for Healthcare Research and Quality, *www.ahrq.gov/qual/psoact.htm*.

 Creating a Just Culture

Planning the Change

- Select strategies to identify stakeholders and champions

- State learning objectives for a just culture staff educational program

Once the culture assessment has been completed, leadership now has the daunting task of looking at what the findings tell them, including what the staff perceives as the organization's problem areas. In many cases, their perceptions are on target, but staff members are also fairly accurate in their assessment of the strengths of the organization. Once leadership has taken a look at what the staff has told them about what they perceive as needing to be changed in the organization to move toward a more just and fair culture, it is up to the administrative team to hear what department managers and staff are saying and to work with them to plan how to begin the change process.

Anticipated Goals of Implementing a Just Culture

Remember that change is hard for the majority of folks. It can be difficult for staff to trust that the organization is moving from a punitive approach to one that is more fair and just. No matter how much planning and communicating is done to prepare for the change, folks will still be leery and mistrustful until they actually see the new, more positive attitude in action. To that end, setting goals that have been developed collaboratively by leadership and staff is essential to the successful transition toward implementation of a just culture.

Obviously, the primary goal for any organization, regardless of culture, is to provide safe, high-quality care—this goal should be at the top of the list. However, there should be additional goals that address specifically what the organization wants to achieve by implementing a new, fairer way to look at medical events. The following are some examples for such goals:

- Every person affiliated with the organization is cognizant and aware of the fact that healthcare is a risky business. Every person understands that there are inherent risks to the provision of care and that, on occasion, there will be mistakes made.

- Every staff member understands that although occasional mistakes will be made, staff should continuously work to identify and control or manage hazards or potential hazards. In fact, in a just culture, folks are actually always looking for ways in which an error could occur so that proactive efforts can be made to prevent errors from happening.

- It is clearly understood that willful or intentional violations of policy or protocol will absolutely not be tolerated.

- Employees and leadership clearly understand and agree on what is acceptable and unacceptable behavior.

- Employees are encouraged to proactively report anything thought to pose a potential safety hazard.

- When hazards or adverse medical events are reported, they are analyzed using an objective method of evaluating why the event occurred. Identified patterns and trends are reviewed and shared with staff, and actions are taken to address them.

- Hazards and medical errors, and actions to control them, are tracked and reported regularly at all levels of the organization.

- Employees, volunteers, contracted individuals, and medical staff are all encouraged to develop and apply their own skills and knowledge to enhance organizational safety. In this case, it's okay to use those critical-thinking skills and consider thinking outside the box to achieve the organization's goals.

- Staff and management feel free to communicate openly and frequently concerning safety hazards, medical errors, potentially compensable events, etc.

- Lessons learned should be discussed openly and regularly following an event occurrence so that leadership and staff can share with others what not to do in the future and also to prevent recurrence of a similar event.

- Feedback regarding reporting and adverse events is provided. Staff are interested in hearing whenever an adverse event is reported and appreciate knowing the outcome of any adverse event, including what actions were taken to address why the event occurred, if there was anything they could have done differently to avert the event's occurrence, etc.[1]

Leverage Current Strengths

Ten years ago at Johns Hopkins Hospital in Baltimore, two patient safety culture assessment survey tools were used—one to assess staff members' perception of where the organization stood with respect to safety as a strategic initiative (otherwise known as a Safety Climate Scale), and one to assess the extent that patient safety was felt to be a strategic initiative at the senior leadership level (otherwise known as a Strategies for Leadership Survey). When findings were analyzed, there were three areas highlighted as opportunities for improving patient safety:

- Senior leaders needed to be more visible to the frontline staff

- Proactive patient safety strategies needed to be put into place

- Physicians needed to become involved with and be educated about patient safety

In other words, these survey findings didn't say folks were doing a bad job providing quality patient care. However, what the results did reflect was a picture of staff's perceptions about whether senior leadership valued them as employees, as people honestly trying to do their best every day, who for whatever reason feel that making and reporting a mistake could very well lead to them feeling punished rather than their behavior objectively being evaluated. Senior leadership needs to take a hard, long look at what the staff identifies as potential barriers to the organization's goal of being a patient-safety-focused organization. This is very valuable feedback that can be incorporated into the overall organizational patient safety strategic plan.

For example, a staff member might identify and bring to the forefront a problem that exists with middle management's inconsistent application of just and fair actions when an employee has committed an error. However, that staff member might also recognize that the hospital is dedicated to doing the right thing by wanting to promote a more just and consistent approach to appropriate error management and perceives human resources leadership as helpful in trying to promote consistent policy application. The hospital then has an obligation to take advantage of the staff member's positive feedback about the human resources department and ask the staff member for his or her assistance in developing policies and procedures that are considered to be fair and that can be applied consistently by all managers (and still meet whatever legal or other regulatory requirements are necessary to satisfy human resources).

When problems are identified, solutions must be developed to specifically target those identified areas in order to be effective in changing behavior and, ultimately, the organization's culture. Because change is being effected via one identified problem at a time, some folks might consider that it is best to make change occur using baby steps rather than attempting to change everything at once. Therefore, hospitals should recognize incremental change as an essential component in moving the organization toward a just culture.

Additionally, hospitals can further promote their move toward a more just culture by educating the community about their desire to improve public perception of how to treat medical errors. The hospital should educate the public on its new methods, which include a more collaborative and open style of managing medical errors. Hospitals can influence and encourage this type of collaborative approach to addressing medical errors (committed by healthcare professionals) by working with state medical and nursing boards, professional associations, the legal and judicial profession, legislative representatives,

 Creating a Just Culture

the media, and other interested parties so that the focus can be on all parties mutually learning from mistakes and educating the public objectively rather than by punitive action for one unintentional act that caused harm and for which those who were involved in the error will forever be affected.

Although the healthcare community should accept responsibility for the fact that the event occurred and ensure its members that appropriate steps are being taken to ensure that the individual accepts responsibility for making the mistake, the organization also needs to communicate very clearly to the community that a thorough evaluation of all related processes will take place to determine which systems or processes had breakdowns that need to be repaired. The hospital needs to communicate that the error most likely occurred because of the breakdown and that, once the breakdown has been repaired, steps will be taken to ensure that the error will not be repeated.

Hospitals should begin to establish relationships with people who have influence over public perceptions and have steps already in place to proactively address a response to the media. Such steps would include being the initiator of the call whenever a serious incident has occurred that has the potential to become a public event. Have medical experts standing by ready to answer any questions and help the community understand how something like this can happen through process or system breakdown, not individual error.

State hospital associations are a wonderful leverage tool because they represent all of their hospital members and can speak on their behalf both individually and as an industry about what the medical community is doing to promote patient safety and prevent patient harm. They also have the ears of many community leaders who may not be medically educated but are upstanding members in their neighborhoods, area banks, schools, civic associations, and other local organizations, groups, and functions, who in turn can continue the healthcare profession's efforts to educate the community about steps being taken to provide high-quality care and keep patients and community members safe while in the hospital's care.

Hospitals and state hospital associations can also communicate with leading authorities in the areas of quality, risk management, and patient safety by tooting their own horns at the national level about the progress they have made within their own communities. A primary example of this is how open, communicative, and responsive Johns Hopkins Children's Center was with the entire family in the aftermath of the death of Josie King, the 18-month-old girl who died in January 2001, after a domino effect of errors led to severe dehydration and a medication overdose, from which she did not recover. The hospital worked with Josie's mother, Sorrel King, and made efforts to develop an honest and open line of communication with her about the progress taking place toward making the hospital a safer place for children. Sorrel and leaders from the hospital spoke at the national level about educating providers and the public about the need to work with those who have committed the errors, evaluate the causes, learn from the old processes, and develop and implement better ones. The hospital also promoted safer practices. As a result of the hospital's openness, more and more hospitals and healthcare providers across the country and around the world are aware of the need for taking a more just approach with staff members when addressing how to manage the unanticipated outcome when a medical error occurs.

Identifying Stakeholders and Champions

Once senior leadership has the information on what make a just culture, what should be done with it? It is then time for raising awareness of the importance of patient safety to the organization, beginning at the top with the board of directors and continuing on down the food chain to frontline staff members. Start by educating key leaders first. In my experience, key leaders including the board members, CEO, chief operating officer, chief nursing officer, chief financial officer, chief risk officer, chief medical officer, and other key clinical leaders, must actively engage in educational sessions that are presented by known experts in the field, like David Marx, Michael Cohen, or Peter Pronovost.

Champions are those folks who are on the side of the patient and are willing to put themselves out on a limb to create change. They are committed to promoting patient safety and preventing patient harm, won't get discouraged easily or give up the fight, and are flexible—they understand that there can be several different ways to achieve the same goal. They are continuously gathering new ideas from others and are willing to go to bat for the patient safety officer's efforts, such as by assisting with staff education about a just and safe culture. These staff members are not afraid to confront leadership when there is conflict about doing what's right, ensuring the organization is committed to a hazard-free, patient-safe healthcare environment. These folks can be members of the board, senior leadership, medical staff, managers, or even frontline staff. Anyone willing to serve as an

Creating a Just Culture

outspoken advocate of patient safety and of a just approach to error management can serve as a champion, and there can be several in an organization.

Once key leaders are on board, they can begin training everyone else in the organization and across the system, starting at the director/manager/supervisor level. This is a good place to start; as one human resources staff member told me during a recent interview about the vital need to have human resources at the table: "If you in any way evaluate the performance or behavior of another individual, you need to attend the training." It absolutely needs to be mandatory for folks at this level.

Topics that need to be emphasized in this training include an overview of the just culture concept, the three classifications of behaviors, why people choose to exhibit the behaviors that they do, and the associated consequences. There should be a good deal of role-playing and, when sessions are completed, leaders should not only have a better understanding of the concept, but they should also realize that this approach is a fairer way of managing the behavior of their staff. This approach is just because it involves coming up with new solutions for handling similar events in the future that are less likely to put patient safety at risk while still holding the employee accountable for his or her actions without being punitive in the approach. It is also more credible to use experts in the field of just culture and patient safety, at least initially, for the training. In most instances, leadership understands and stands behind the results: safer patients in their hospitals.

Once the management team has been trained, the organization can choose to go in either of the following directions. The first is to educate the entire staff about the move toward a just culture within the organization so that everyone has a clear understanding of the new expectations and will learn that patient safety is of significant importance to leadership; the second approach requires managers to begin assimilating what they have learned into their own managerial style, incorporating these techniques and applying them in their everyday management activities, and including these principles in new-employee orientation and routine educational sessions. In other words, this approach is about managers walking the walk and talking the talk. By leading by example, the culture changes. It's what staff members will take stock in—while most hospital staff members look to leadership in a parental way, they look at these managers as people to emulate.

The second approach exists because staff may have a cynical perception of leadership. For the past 20–30 years, generally speaking, staff members' perceptions have been that leadership's main focus is always on the financial aspects of the organization. To that end, they have been skeptical of leadership's true motives for years and only when or if they see the change with their own eyes are they likely to believe that the new culture being exhibited by leadership really is a just one and that leadership truly does support just concepts.

However, it's worth noting (and teaching staff) that the financial bottom line and increased patient safety are not always forces driving against one another. Oftentimes there is a tremendous reduction in the number of adverse events when an organization has created a "positive reinforcement culture" of safe behaviors and disciplinary systems that allow employees to come forward and report their mistakes. Studies also show that prompt and full disclosure to patients and families about an adverse event, accepting appropriate responsibility and communicating with openness and honesty, has led to a reduction in medical malpractice claims and settlements.

An example of the potential power of an open and just culture can be seen in the case of Michael Woods, brother of actor James Woods, who died from the alleged failure to diagnose an impending heart attack as a result of negligent treatment by the emergency department of Kent County Hospital in Warwick, RI, in 2006. For the two years leading up to the trial, and the first three weeks of the trial itself, no one from the hospital had ever spoken to the family regarding what had happened to Michael and the circumstances surrounding his death, which was the reason the Woods' family filed the lawsuit in the first place. According to the hospital CEO, Sandra Coletta, the Woods family's demeanor was angry and bitter during the trial and it was at this point she realized that no one from the hospital had ever spoken to them about the event, nor had anyone ever apologized for the event occurring. As soon as Coletta went to speak to the family, the manner exhibited by members of the Woods family changed completely and, after further discussion, both sides announced the withdrawal of the lawsuit and that a fair settlement had been reached, with James Woods praising Coletta for personally coming to them.

Furthermore, Woods stated that the impetus for settlement was a phone call from Coletta the night before the lawsuit was actually withdrawn, saying she was sorry for his family's loss.

 Creating a Just Culture

He said it was the first time anyone from the hospital had initiated communication with them, and that to him and the rest of his family, it made all the difference in the world and led to them wanting to get this issue resolved. Additionally, the hospital agreed to contribute $1.25 million toward the establishment of the Michael Woods Patient Safety Institute, a center dedicated to research relating to and education about improving and promoting patient safety efforts and bringing them to the public's attention.[2]

Develop a Just Culture Principle Document

A just culture principle document, like the one developed by the Dana-Farber Cancer Institute (see Figure 3.1), in essence articulates quite clearly the organization's commitment to ensuring that a just culture is deeply valued by the organization and describes the components of the just culture principle, such as education, consistency, communication, and commitment to continuous performance improvement and patient safety. This document needs to be shared throughout the organization and incorporated into every aspect of daily operations, reflected in the preface of every policy and procedure, and communicated at every educational opportunity, in both formal presentations as well as informally at town meetings, during walk-arounds, and whenever the opportunity presents itself, leaving no doubt of its importance to those most responsible for ensuring that the just culture principle is a true strategic priority.

Implementing New, Fair, and Just Policies and Procedures

The next step is to develop new policies and procedures to follow your organization's new way of thinking, as well as to get rid of the ones that no longer apply.

For example, you should check whether your hospital has:

- A formalized policy and procedure for reporting adverse events

- Staff awareness of the types of events that should be reported

- A standardized taxonomy to which your staff can refer if they need guidance or a written description of what types of events should be reported

FIGURE 3.1

Dana-Farber Cancer Institute principles of a fair and just culture

Background

It is inevitable that people will make mistakes or experience misunderstandings in any work environment. When events occur that cause harm or have the potential to cause harm to patients or staff members, or that place the Institute at legal, financial, or ethical risk, a choice exists: to learn or to blame. Dana-Farber Cancer Institute is committed to creating a work environment that emphasizes learning rather than blame.

Dana-Farber Cancer Institute recognizes the complexity and interdependence of the work environment in all aspects of its operations, including patient care, clinical operations, research, support services, and administration. The intent is to promote an atmosphere where any employee can openly discuss errors of commission or omission, process improvements, and/or systems corrections without the fear of reprisal.

It is well documented that most errors, whether or not they cause harm, are due to breakdowns in organizational systems; however, when an error takes place, individual culprits are often sought. Blaming individuals creates a culture of fear and defensiveness that diminishes both learning and the capacity to constantly improve systems.

Most errors take place within systems that themselves contribute to the error. In spite of this, it is difficult to create an institutional culture that integrates the understanding that systems failures are the root cause of most errors. Learning from errors often points to beneficial changes in systems and management processes as well as in individual behavior.

In the context of promoting a fair and just culture, what does it mean? A fair and just culture means giving constructive feedback and critical analysis in skillful ways, doing assessments that are based on facts, and having respect for the complexity of the situation. It also means providing fair-minded treatment, having productive conversations, and creating effective structures that help people reveal their errors and help the organization learn from them. A fair and just culture does <u>not</u> mean non-accountable, nor does it mean an avoidance of critique or assessment of competence. Rather, when incompetence or sub-standard performance is revealed after careful collection of facts, and/or there is reckless or willful violation of policies or negligent behavior, corrective or disciplinary action may be appropriate.

Applying these principles creates an opportunity to enact the core values of the Dana-Farber Cancer Institute. In order to have the greatest impact and achieve the highest level of excellence, staff must be able to speak up about problems, errors, conflicts and misunderstandings in an environment where it is the shared goal to identify and discuss problems with curiosity and respect. To achieve excellence, unwanted or unexpected outcomes and inefficiencies of practice must be used as the basis for a learning process. Respect must be shown to all people at every level of the organization.

 Creating a Just Culture

Dana-Farber Cancer Institute principles of a fair and just culture (cont.)

1. DFCI strives to create a learning environment and a workplace that support the core values of impact, excellence, respect/compassion and discovery in every aspect of work at the Institute.

2. DFCI supports the efforts of every individual to deliver the best work possible. When errors are made and/or misunderstandings occur, the Institute strives to establish accountability in the context of the system in which they occurred.

   ➤ We commit to creating an institutional work environment that is least likely to cause or support error.
   ➤ We are proactive about identifying system flaws.

3. DFCI commits to holding individuals accountable for their own performance in accordance with their job responsibilities and the DFCI core values. However, individuals should not carry the burden for system flaws over which they had no control.

4. DFCI promotes open interdisciplinary discussion of untoward events (errors, mistakes, misunderstandings, or system failures resulting in harm, potential harm, or adverse outcome) by all who work, visit, or are cared for at the Institute.

   ➤ We commit to developing and maintaining easily available and simple processes to discuss untoward events.
   ➤ We commit to eliciting different points of view to identify sources of untoward events and to use the information to improve the working and care environment.
   ➤ We commit to fostering an interdisciplinary teamwork approach to the analysis of untoward events and to the actions taken to address them.
   ➤ We believe that individuals are responsible for surfacing untoward events and for contributing to the elimination of system flaws.
   ➤ We commit to analyzing episodes of institutional or patient harm or potential harm in an unbiased fashion to best determine the contributions of system and individual factors.
   ➤ We seek solutions that promote simplification and standardization wherever possible.

5. DFCI acts to improve all areas of the workplace by implementing changes based on our analysis of problems and potential or actual harm.

   ➤ We know that actions designed to address the root causes of untoward events will improve the effectiveness of our work environment and the safety of care. We commit to identifying and assigning responsibility for implementing those actions to specific individuals or groups.
   ➤ We commit to developing timely and effective follow-up and an effective organizational culture through education and systems for ensuring on-going competency.

6. DFCI commits to a culture of inclusion and education.

   ➤ We commit to fostering a culture that is concerned with safety in research, clinical care and administration through continuous education, proactive interventions, and safety-based leadership.
   ➤ We believe that patient input is indispensable to the delivery of safe care and we commit to promoting patient and family participation.

7. DFCI will assess our success in promoting a learning environment by evaluating our willingness to communicate openly and by the improvements we achieve.

   ➤ We commit to monitoring actions and attitudes for their effectiveness in supporting a culture of safety and modifying actions as needed.

[Principles adapted from Allan Frankel, M.D. and the Patient Safety Leaders at Partners Healthcare System]

Source: Dana-Farber Cancer Institute, Boston.

Suppose a medical mistake occurred that was fairly obvious, put the patient at some risk, and required medical intervention to stabilize the patient; or, more specifically, suppose the patient was administered penicillin despite the fact that there was significant documentation in the medical record as well as on the patient's hospital room door indicating that he or she is severely allergic to the drug. The patient developed an acute anaphylactic reaction that required the immediate administration of epinephrine, steroids, antihistamines, etc., to counteract the reaction in order to stabilize him or her and the patient was transferred to the intensive care unit for close, 24-hour, one-to-one nursing observation. The ultimate outcome is that there is no long-term consequence; the patient will ultimately be fine. However, clearly two things need to happen: First, the error needs to be reported to the supervisor of the unit on which the error occurred, as well as to risk or quality management, and second, the patient and the patient's family need to be made aware of the event.

The disclosure of an adverse event needs to be done in a manner that is nonaccusatory, objective, straightforward, and nonblaming. The family needs to be made aware of what actions will be taken to ensure that a similar event does not happen to someone else in the future, but just as importantly, the staff need to see that this approach does not place blame on anyone in particular, and that what is being described is a summary of the facts as they occurred and what was done for the patient the minute the event was discovered.

Continuing with the same example, suppose that after the event occurred the patient was doing well and had been transferred back to the regular floor. Once the patient was settled into his or her new room, he or she was instructed per the doctor's orders not to get out of bed without assistance. Staff leave the room to take care of another patient and after a bit, the patient uses the call bell to ask for some help getting to the bathroom, but had to wait for more than an hour before someone acknowledges the call and provides assistance, causing the patient to be very upset. The patient wants to voice a complaint. Staff need to know the process for allowing the patient to submit a grievance or complaint, and carry out that process promptly and correctly.

To ensure that there is consistent reporting of an incident to the appropriate individuals, you need a policy in place for reporting, disclosing, and filing grievances. A sample of such a policy can be found in Figure 3.2. There must be a known, consistent process with respect to how the disclosure of information to the patient and/or family about an adverse event and when the disclosure should take place. Your incident reporting policy, patient grievance/complaint policy, and your disclosure policy should include the following components:

- Definitions of specific terms

- Process for filing a patient grievance/complaint

- How and by whom patient complaints and grievances will be investigated

- How patient complaint/grievance data will be used as lessons learned for staff

- How and how often patient complaint/grievance data will be reported to individual departments, appropriate committees, senior leadership, and the board of trustees

- Purpose of incident reporting

- Who should report an incident

- The procedure for reporting an incident

- Who is responsible for investigating the incident

- How incident report data is utilized to promote patient safety and prevent patient harm (e.g., analysis for pattern and trend identification)

- Under what circumstances employees will be held accountable for learning from their mistakes when reporting nonintentional or nonmalicious events, as well as when disciplinary action would be necessary (e.g., failing to report an event, causing deliberate harm, etc.)

- How, to whom, and how often incident report data is reported to individual departments, appropriate committees, senior leadership, and the board of directors

- The definition of the types of events that should be disclosed (organization-specific)

- To whom the disclosure should be made

- When disclosure should take place

FIGURE
3.2

Incident reporting administrative policy

TITLE: INCIDENT REPORTING POLICY – COMPLAINT/GRIEVANCE REPORTING
ORIGINAL ISSUE DATE:

I. PURPOSE

To ensure that all incidents not consistent with the routine operations of the hospital or the routine care of a particular patient are reported to the Quality Management Department so that immediate attention and responses can be given to individual occurrences. Statistics can then be derived from the collective number of incidents reported and will serve as a basis for adverse patient trends, patient safety issues, or other risks and hazards to be identified, and risk reduction programs implemented.

In order to promote a culture that promotes patient safety, the hospital's Incident Reporting Policy is based upon a nonpunitive approach to incident/occurrence reporting. The hospital leadership will encourage open and honest reporting of injuries and hazards to patients, visitors, and staff, and this process will be nonpunitive in nature for all persons reporting incidents throughout the organization. Incidence/occurrence investigations will be viewed as an opportunity for education and/or process improvement, and will focus on processes and systems, rather than human error.

Disciplinary action will be limited to only those employees who engage in willful or malicious misconduct, or those occurrences in which the employee failed to report an incident or hazard to patients in a timely manner.

II. INCIDENT REPORTING ADMINISTRATIVE POLICY
RESPONSIBILITY

A. All hospital employees, medical staff members, volunteers, and contract service members will participate in the hospitalwide incident reporting program. All incidents such as those listed as follows will be reported to the Department of Quality Management:

1. Incidents involving inconsistencies with written hospital policies and procedures (e.g., informed consent, bedrails, patient restraints, nursing/physician professional relationships, confidential patient information released to the public, etc.)

2. Unanticipated and nonroutine employee, contract service personnel, patient, visitor, and volunteer injuries resulting from accidents or errors such as: falls for any reason, with or without injuries; medication errors; needle punctures and/or occupational exposures; diagnostic/therapeutic procedures performed on wrong patients; burns from heating pads; x-rays; broken teeth; pressure sores; etc.

Creating a Just Culture

Incident reporting administrative policy (cont.)

3. Mishaps due to faulty/defective equipment or adverse conditions in our physical facility. (Refer to Safe Medical Device Act Policy for reporting of faulty/defective medical equipment.)

4. Sudden, unexpected adverse results of professional care and treatment, death; brain damage; physical, mental, or emotional loss or impairment; cardiac/respiratory arrests; or any occurrence or situation that necessitates additional hospitalization or a dramatic change in patient treatment regimens.

5. All vocal or written expressions of dissatisfaction from the patient or patient families concerning the professional and nonprofessional services.

6. All incidents involving patient, employee, visitor, or volunteer property claimed to be lost, stolen, or damaged.

B. The Quality Management Department will review, investigate, and apply risk management protocols to the incidents reported in accord with its departmental policy and procedures.

C. The Quality Management Department will collect, maintain, and distribute statistical data to specific committees from information generated from the collective total submission of incidents reported. This data can be utilized to identify adverse trends in patient and environmental safety, in order to facilitate continuous improvement and maximize safety for patients, employees, volunteers, and visitors.

D. It will be the individual responsibility of the employee to know and follow all policies and procedures associated with his or her assigned duties, use sound judgment and awareness of potential hazards before taking action, and promptly report incidents/occurrences.

E. Management will be responsible for educating staff regarding the reporting of incidents/occurrences and continuing performance improvement regarding patient safety, involving the staff in the investigative process to identify system and process deficiencies along with performance-improvement activities, and focusing on the "how" and "why" of an incident, rather than "who" may have been involved or contributed to it.

Management will also be responsible for establishing the culture that promotes incident occurrence reporting in a nonpunitive environment, and implementing corrective action plans where necessary in order to reduce risk to patients, visitors, and staff.

F. Administrative and Medical Staff will be responsible for promoting the culture of nonpunitive reporting by encouraging reporting, while avoiding blaming those involved. They will also be responsible for providing for the continuing education of physicians regarding safety issues and practices, and report any incidents/ occurrences they may be aware of.

FIGURE
3.2

Incident reporting administrative policy (cont.)

G. The Board of Trustees will receive and monitor ongoing risk management and safety information/data at least annually, and allocate appropriate resources to support the program.

H. No employee, staff member, volunteer, or contract service member will be subject to disciplinary action for reporting unintentional or non-malicious incidents. Employees will be subject to disciplinary action and/or employment termination for failure to report known incidents or occurrences.

III. PROCEDURE

A. INCIDENT REPORTS

1. Incident reports of all types, including Patient/Visitor Fall Incident Reports, Medication Error Incident Reports, Adverse Drug Event/IV Infiltration Incident Reports, Equipment Malfunction Incident Reports, and General Miscellaneous Incident Reports, are to be initiated and completed in their entirety by the hospital employee, staff member, volunteer, or contract service member directly involved in, responding to, or involved in the discovery of incurred incidents.

2. The supervisor or designee is responsible for the initial investigation of the incident, such as identifying witnesses or safety negligence issues due to falls, occupational exposures, injury, etc.

3. Written incident reports are to be signed by both the individual preparing the report and the department head or designee and should reach the risk manager within a timely manner. Serious incidents should be reported immediately to the risk manager with written incident report follow-up.

4. The Quality Management Department, in accord with established departmental criteria and individual fact situations, shall facilitate investigation and preserve for reference and use the information obtained through medical records review, witness interviews, defective equipment/supplies, and any other applicable data.

5. All incidents considered by the risk manager to be potentially compensable will be reported to applicable casualty insurance companies.

6. Statistical data generated from the information derived from the collective submission of incident reports will be reported to the Quality Review Committee as reflected in the Bylaws and to Administration and the Board of Trustees annually, or when requested. Statistical data will also be referred to the appropriate Patient Safety Committees.

FIGURE
3.2

Incident reporting administrative policy (cont.)

7. The Quality Management Department will recommend and otherwise work with the entire hospital community in applying applicable risk treatment processes in order to enhance the quality of professional patient care services and prevent and/or reduce the frequency and severity of employee, patient, staff member, visitor, volunteer, or contract service personnel injury and liability situations.

8. Concerning the reporting of incidents/occurrences, employees are not subject to disciplinary action EXCEPT as follows:

    a. An event is not reported in a timely fashion.

    b. Event involves sabotage, malicious behavior, chemical impairment, or criminal activity.

    c. False information is provided on the Incident Report or in follow-up investigation.

    d. An employee fails to respond to educational efforts and/or fails to participate in the education or other preventive plan.

9. Employees who meet any of the exceptions listed in section #8 above will be subject to disciplinary action in accordance with Human Resources policy and procedures.

10. All employees, patients, staff members, visitors, volunteers, and contract service personnel who sustain bodily injury in an incident will be offered medical attention. An incident report should be completed by any employee or nonemployee (patients, visitors, volunteers, or contract service personnel) at the time of treatment if not already completed or as soon as possible if the injury is serious. If treatment is refused, a single statement to that effect should be completed. If the person refuses to sign, a notation of that effect will be made on the incident report.

    • FOR EMPLOYEES' INJURIES ONLY: Refer to Section 5.6 of the Personnel Policy Manual for the policy and procedure regarding reporting and management of Employee Injuries. Injury packets will be available to injured employees either from their supervisor, Occupational Health, Emergency Department, Human Resources, or Employee Health. Employees will be asked to complete the Ohio Bureau of Workers' Compensation First Report of Injury Report (FROI) and the Employee Injury/ Occurrence Form.

    • FOR VOLUNTEERS ONLY: Personal insurance will be billed first. The hospital will write off any remaining balance for the initial treatment only. Each case will need to be individually considered by the risk manager and/or the CEO with regard to any further payment of incurred charges.

FIGURE
3.2

Incident reporting administrative policy (cont.)

- MOBILE MEALS VOLUNTEERS ONLY: Personal insurance will be billed first for personal injury. The hospital will then write off any remaining balance for the initial treatment only. Each case will need to be individually considered by the risk manager and/or the CEO with regard to any further payment of incurred charges. In regards to auto damage, refer to the Volunteers' Policy and Procedure book.

- VISITORS/PATIENTS ONLY: Personal insurance will be billed first. The hospital will consider the write-off of any remaining balance, up to 20% of the total charges, for the initial treatment only. Each case will need to be individually considered by the risk manager and/or the CEO with regard to any further payment of incurred charges.

- CONTRACT SERVICE PERSONNEL ONLY: The employing entity will be billed as an industrial claim.

B.   UNANTICIPATED OUTCOMES

Patients and, when appropriate, their families are informed about the outcomes of care, including unanticipated outcomes. The intent is that the responsible licensed independent practitioner or designee should clearly explain the outcome of any treatment or procedure to the patient and family when appropriate, whenever those outcomes differ significantly from the anticipated outcomes of care.

1.   Patients and, when appropriate, their families must be informed about outcomes of care that the patient (or family) must be knowledgeable about in order to participate in current and future decisions affecting the patient's care, and

2.   Unanticipated outcomes of care that relate to sentinel events considered reviewable by The Joint Commission. The responsible licensed independent practitioner or his or her designee informs the patient (and when appropriate, the patient's family) about these outcomes of care.

There may be, on occasion, an appropriate situation that justifies nondisclosure of an unanticipated outcome. An example would be if the disclosure would cause psychological harm, or further complicate the patient's medical condition. The decision not to disclose an unanticipated outcome would be made by the physician in conjunction with Risk Management. Risk Management should document the reason for nondisclosure.

Definition of Unanticipated Outcome — A result that differs significantly from what was anticipated to be the result of a treatment or procedure.

                                           Creating a Just Culture

FIGURE 3.2 | **Incident reporting administrative policy (cont.)**

PURPOSE

- To address the issue of unanticipated outcomes

- To describe how and when unanticipated outcomes are disclosed to patients and, when appropriate, their families

- To educate physicians and staff on the disclosure of unanticipated outcomes

SEVERITY OF EVENT

For the purposes of disclosure of unanticipated outcomes, the following grading system is utilized:

- Level 1: An event occurred but the patient was not harmed

- Level 2: An event occurred that resulted in the need for increased patient assessment/monitoring, but there was no change in vital signs and no patient harm

- Level 3: An event occurred that resulted in the need for treatment and/or intervention and caused temporary patient harm

- Level 4: An event occurred that resulted in initial or prolonged hospitalization, and caused temporary patient harm

- Level 5: An event occurred that resulted in permanent patient harm or a near-death event, such as anaphylaxis

- Level 6: An event occurred that resulted in patient death

DISCLOSURE

1. What events should be disclosed?

   - Disclosure of unanticipated outcomes should be performed in occurrences that are scored a Level of Severity (see above) from 3 to 6. For example, this would include an unexpected admission to intensive care, unexpected patient death, returns to the OR, wrong-site surgery, or a medication error that results in death or patient harm.

   - Errors that do not harm patients and do not have the potential to do so (insignificant or minor incidents) do not require disclosure to the patient. If there is a question concerning disclosure, contact the Risk Management Department.

FIGURE
3.2

Incident reporting administrative policy (cont.)

2. To whom should disclosure be made?

    - Disclosure of unanticipated outcomes should be made to the patient and, when appropriate, the patient's family or personal representative (i.e., parent, guardian, durable power of attorney).

3. When should disclosure take place?

    - Disclosure of unanticipated outcomes should take place as soon as practical after the event has been identified. Disclosure to the patient should occur when the patient is stable and/or able to comprehend the information. Disclosure to the patient's family or personal representative may occur sooner depending on the incident's severity and his/her need to know this information.

4. Who should disclose events to patients?

    - Prior to disclosure, the physician and the appropriate department manager will consult with Risk Management regarding what should be disclosed and how disclosure is made. There are several ways in which an unexpected outcome may be disclosed, depending on the event. In some circumstances further investigation may be required to determine which individual(s) should be involved. The attending physician and the risk manager will consider involving representatives from nursing, allied health professionals, pastoral care, social workers, or staff members known to and trusted by the patient/family.

    If the attending physician is unwilling or unable to disclose the event after consultation with Risk Management, or if investigation determines that his or her involvement could exacerbate the problem, the risk manager will work with administration to identify the appropriate person to handle this responsibility.

5. How should disclosure occur?

    - The nature, severity, and cause (if known) of the unexpected outcome should be presented in a straightforward and nonjudgmental fashion. An expression of sorrow is often appropriate and not an admission of guilt. Speculation should be avoided and focus placed on what is known at the time of the discussion. Answer questions and provide assurance that unanswered questions will be investigated further. Describe what, if anything, can be done to correct the consequences of the unanticipated outcome.

FIGURE
3.2

Incident reporting administrative policy (cont.)

6. How is disclosure documented?

- Relevant information on the unanticipated outcome should be documented in the medical record. A summary of the disclosure should be documented in the medical record. This documentation should include:

    1. Documentation of the time, date, and place that disclosure took place;

    2. The name and relationships of those present;

    3. Documentation in appropriate cases that as further information becomes available, this information will be shared with the patient and, when appropriate, his or her personal representative;

    4. Documentation of an offer to be of assistance and the response to it;

    5. Documentation of any questions posed by the patient, family, or legally authorized representative, and the answers provided by the caregiver; and

    6. In specific cases in which a decision is made to withhold some or all information, appropriate documentation is made of the reason(s) for this decision.

- It is acknowledged that in some cases the documentation may be separate from the medical record to protect the safety or welfare of the patient or to prevent interference in law enforcement investigations.

Reference:

1. Joint Commission Standard RI.1.2.2
2. AMA Code of Medical Ethics, Section 8.12
3. ASHRM, Perspectives on Disclosure of Unanticipated Outcome Information
4. Anticipating Unanticipated Outcomes, Client Bulletin, Bricker & Eckler LLP, Aug. 17, 2001

IV. ROUTING

Incidents are reported directly from the floor to the department head, unit supervisor, or designee, who then routes the reports directly to the Quality Management Department in a timely manner.

Statistical incident report information and data will be regularly provided to all appropriate departments, the Quality Review Committee, Safety Committee, and the Joint Conference Committee by the Quality Management/ Risk Management Department.

FIGURE
3.2

Incident reporting administrative policy (cont.)

V. GENERAL

Incident reports are never to be filed in patient or employee records. It is not to be documented in the patient's medical record that an incident report has been completed.

Hospital employees, contract service personnel, staff members, and volunteers are not to discuss the circumstances surrounding incidents with, or in the presence of, patients, visitors, or other outside hospital sources.

Incident reports are to be completed factually, objectively, legibly, and without extraneous comments based on personal opinion, conjecture, or editorial comments.

For confidentiality purposes, incident reports are never to be photocopied, duplicated, or posted by anyone other than the risk manager or at his/her direction.

Incident reports shall not contain recommendations or comments for disciplinary action.

Incident reports shall contain only factual information.

Incident reports may contain indications of corrective action in cases of equipment failure, removal of environmental hazards, or corrective patient care activity.

In the event that behavioral health patients are involved in "major unusual incidents," such as suicide, elopement with injury, altercations with significant injury, overdose, or self-mutilation, these MUST BE reported to the Ohio Department of Mental Health. Contact Risk Management or Legal Services for assistance with reporting.

VI. EMPLOYEE INJURY REPORTING

OBJECTIVE

1. To ensure that all employee incidents/injuries are reported and appropriate medical care and/or follow-up testing is provided in a timely manner.

2. To enable Memorial Hospital to investigate each incident/injury in an attempt to prevent future incidents and reduce future risks.

POLICY

All employees involved in a work-related incident with or without bodily injury will be offered medical attention. Refer to Section 5.6: Workers' Compensation in the hospital personnel policy manual for detailed information regarding roles and responsibilities in the employee incident-reporting process. All employees sustaining a work-related injury will complete a BWC First Report of Injury and an Employee Incident/Occurrence Form. After initial treatment or refusal of treatment (immediately after the incident), the Employee Incident/Occurrence Form will be

FIGURE
3.2

Incident reporting administrative policy (cont.)

forwarded to the Safety Director, who will facilitate any required investigation of the incident with the employee's department manager. The Safety Director, in conjunction with the department manager, will complete and forward this investigation report to the Quality Management/Risk Management Department. A summary and statistical report of all employee injuries will be reported to the Safety and Quality Review Committees on a monthly basis. All incident reports and investigative documentation records will be maintained in the Quality Management/Risk Management offices.

VII. COMPLAINT/GRIEVANCE REVIEW

All vocal or written expressions of dissatisfaction from patients or patients' families, questions of appropriateness of care, etc., concerning the professional and nonprofessional services will be addressed by the risk manager or designee.

1. The employee/physician who receives the complaint or witnesses the occurrence initiates the "Complaint/Grievance Occurrence Review" form by completing the complaint statement.

2. This form is then referred to the Quality Management Department, who will then facilitate the subsequent investigation and involve the various department managers/supervisors, if applicable.

3. The complainant may be contacted by the appropriate manager for clarification or for additional information concerning the complaint.

A. GRIEVANCE INVESTIGATION AND REPORTING

Definition:

Grievance: A "grievance" is a formal, complaint that is filed by a patient when an issue cannot be resolved promptly by staff present. A grievance may be filed verbally or in writing.

Investigation of any formal grievance concerning professional or nonprofessional services will be addressed by the Quality Management/Risk Management (QM/RM) Department or designee. This process has been delegated to the QM/RM Department by the hospital Board of Trustees.

1. According to CMS Conditions of Participation Standards, section 482.13, a hospital must inform each patient (or his or her representative) of the patient's right to file a grievance in advance of furnishing or discontinuing care. Patients must be informed of whom to contact to file a grievance.

2. The employee/physician who receives the formal grievance (verbal or written) will immediately contact the QM/RM Department or the Administration Office to initiate the investigation.

FIGURE

3.2

Incident reporting administrative policy (cont.)

3. The QM/RM Department will facilitate the subsequent investigation(s) or action(s), which may be needed to involve the various department managers/supervisors if applicable.

4. The complainant may be contacted by the appropriate department manager for clarification or for additional information concerning the grievance.

5. Upon decision of a course of action, the complainant will be contacted by the QM/RM Department or designee by telephone or in writing to communicate the decision. This notice will include the steps taken to investigate the grievance, the results of the grievance investigation process, and the date of completion.

6. All grievances will be investigated promptly and an initial decision reached within 10 business days, unless special investigation is required, which may result in an extension as necessary. Grievances involving situations or practices that place patients in immediate danger will be investigated as quickly as possible.

7. Patients have the right to file their grievance directly with the State agency should they wish, regardless of whether they have first used the hospital's grievance process. Patients may be directed to contact the Quality Review Department for a list of agencies to which they may file their grievance.

8. Medicare beneficiary patients have the right to request a peer review organization (PRO) evaluation of their grievance. MHUC is not mandated to automatically refer Medicare beneficiary grievances to the PRO, but will cooperate fully with the PRO evaluation should the patient request a review.

9. Grievance investigations and outcomes data will be shared monthly in Quality Review meetings in order to determine any potential performance improvement activities that may be necessitated by reported grievances.

This Incident Reporting Administrative Policy was adopted and recommended to the Board by the Quality Review Committee.

Approved by:

Board of Trustees

President, Medical Staff

President, CEO

VP, Medical Affairs

VP, Quality Management

Reprinted with permission from Premier, Inc, www.premierinc.com.

 Creating a Just Culture

- Who should disclose and/or be present during the disclosure

- How disclosure should take place

- How the disclosure should be documented and where

The ECRI Institute has a wonderful sample of both an Incident Reporting Policy as well as a Disclosure Policy, and both can be found in their *Healthcare Risk Control Manual.*

Additionally, you will need to review the medical staff policies and procedures, rules and regulations, and their bylaws so that any reference to punishment is removed, replacing that former emphasis with the principles of accountability and responsibility. The American Medical Association encourages the inclusion of a medical staff code of ethics as part of its bylaws, which should include the following:

- Definitions of certain behaviors

- Types of conduct: appropriate, inappropriate, disruptive

- Interventions

- Procedure for reporting adverse physician behavior

- Non-retaliatory requirements

- Promoting awareness of the medical staff code of ethics to medial staff and the community[3]

You will also need to look at your contractor, volunteer, and student policies and procedures and revise them accordingly.

A checklist of items to be reviewed in policies can be found in Figure 3.3. In particular, staff and patient education should be carefully reviewed. Additionally, the Association of Perioperative Nurses has a wonderful just culture toolkit that includes a terrific staff education module (*www.aorn.org*).

FIGURE 3.3 — Checklist for reviewing policies

The next step is to develop new policies and procedures to follow your organization's new way of thinking, and get rid of the ones that no longer apply. Include a review of the **medical staff policies and procedures, rules and regulations**, and their **bylaws** so that any reference to punishment is removed, replacing that former emphasis with the principles of accountability and responsibility. You will also need to look at your contractor, volunteer, and student policies and procedures and revise them accordingly.

Additional policies to be reviewed and/or included are:

- Adverse-Event Reporting

Reviewed?	Area of focus:
	Taxonomy
	Definitions of types of events reported
	How to complete an accurate report
	How the report is submitted
	Who should report and to whom it should be submitted
	How to document follow-up action
	How to maximize protection from discovery, etc.

- Patient Complaint/Grievance Process

Reviewed?	Area of focus:
	How and by whom patient grievances are handled
	Who should be notified
	Required documentation
	Reporting requirements to licensing and regulatory bodies

- Leadership Education

Reviewed?	Area of focus:
	What is involved in the process
	How the patient safety culture assessment will be administered
	How long it will take to complete the patient safety culture assessment
	How often assessment will be repeated
	Resources required to administer assessment

Creating a Just Culture

Educating staff about new policies

As you develop your own staff educational programs, there are several essential learning objectives for a successful program on a just and safety-focused culture, including:

- Staff understand the human factors associated with errors, and the kind of environment most conducive to error occurrence and error prevention

- Staff understand the three different types of behaviors (human error, at-risk, and reckless) and the consequences associated with each one

- Staff understand that the organization takes a nonpunitive approach to unintentional acts that lead to errors, but will not tolerate willful or intentional acts that lead to harm

- Staff members understand that the organization supports a reporting culture and that they are expected to report their errors and near misses

- Staff understand that leadership encourages a proactive approach to error prevention through vigilance, volunteering to help design safer systems, making safer choices, and following established policies and procedures

- Staff members understand that it is expected they will learn from their mistakes and not make the same ones twice

Staff education can be provided in a variety of ways, but to get the best bang for your buck, case scenarios, role-playing, and training videos are quite effective in getting staff to understand why the organization is moving to a more just approach to addressing medical errors.

I would also encourage folks who are interested in learning more about just culture and patient safety to use the following resources for research or help:

- Local, state, or regional hospital association

- Local patient safety organization

- Josie King Foundation (*www.JosieKingFoundation.org*)

- The Just Culture Community (*www.justculture.org*)

- American Society for Healthcare Risk Management (*www.ashrm.org*)

- National Association for Healthcare Quality (*www.nahq.org*)

- Institute for Safe Medication Practices (*www.ismp.org*)

- Institute for Healthcare Improvement (*www.ihi.org*)

- National Patient Safety Foundation (*www.npsf.org*)

- Agency for Healthcare Research and Quality (*www.ahrq.gov*)

- National Quality Forum (*www.qualityforum.org*)

It's important to include all staff members in this education and to identify champions to role-model good behavior. Figure 3.4 provides a checklist to ensure you are adequately educating your staff.

Educating patients about new policies

Patient education is also crucial to your culture. Be sure the patient and/or family feel that they have a responsibility to be an active participant. Patients should definitely be able to identify any deviation in care and ask questions about care that is being performed in an unfamiliar or improper manner. For example, a patient should always be comfortable asking the caregiver to wash his or her hands before any physical examination takes place. Another way a patient should be actively involved is to question whenever a new medication is being administered. The patient should be sure to ask what it is, what it is supposed to treat, how it is supposed to react to the condition for which it's prescribed, the signs and symptoms of any adverse reactions, and any possible side effects. He or she should always question if a medication looks different than expected and always have prompt access to the primary care provider if there are any questions at all about any medications or the treatment regimen.

 Creating a Just Culture

FIGURE
3.4

Staff education steps and checklist

When training with staff, don't forget to include:

- Medical staff

- Students

- Volunteers

- Contracted or agency personnel

Education should be administered at new-employee orientation and routinely scheduled competency evaluations. Take into account:

- The definition of adverse events

- The reporting of events and by whom they are reported

- The reporting of patient/family complaints

- Potentially compensable events

Identify a patient safety champion. He or she should exhibit:

- A true passion for wanting to do everything possible to provide high-quality care in as safe a manner as possible

- A willingness to learn as much as possible about an effective patient safety culture in order to ensure patient safety

- A desire to share enthusiasm and knowledge with coworkers, patients, and families, as well as with members of the community

Utilize your patient safety champion. He or she should:

- Serve as a patient safety team leader and resource for staff and other members of the healthcare team, patients, and family members

- Be able to provide any additional patient safety information as requested, or at least know where and how to start searching for the requested information

In 2002, the Joint Commission launched its Speak Up™ campaign, which was initiated to encourage patient participation in their own healthcare activities. Today The Joint Commission standards require hospitals not only to provide education to patients and families in an understandable format, but also to incorporate acknowledgment that this teaching actually took place by ensuring that it has been documented in the patient's medical record.

Leadership walk-arounds are also important. In many cases, staff members feel that leadership has been woefully inadequate in its understanding of what frontline staff members have identified as serious quality-of-care concerns as a result of being in the trenches of hands-on patient care. Generally speaking, another bone of contention is usually that leadership is not in touch with the staff's real world. In many cases, staff members report in patient safety culture assessments that leadership doesn't support patient safety efforts that are trying to be made.

A just culture hospital also shares its best practices and other shared learning so that other organizations can learn from one hospital's mistakes and prevent similar events from occurring in their hospitals. If the hospital has a success story using a best practice, this is a great opportunity for it to share its lessons learned and offer the same tools and techniques to its sister hospitals so a more standardized approach is developed within a region and error prevention can be maximized.

The Agency for Healthcare Research and Quality *(www.ahrq.gov)* has a host of tools to help organizations not only get started with measuring their current patient safety culture but also to continue to measure their improvements along what I consider to be an exciting but continuous journey toward a just culture.

References

1. GAIN Working Group E. *A Roadmap to a Just Culture: Enhancing the Safety Environment.* Flight Ops/ATC Ops Safety Information Sharing, 2004.

2. Moore, Russell J. and Howell, John. "4 words led to settlement of Woods' case against Kent," Warwick Beacon, 2009, *www.warwickonline.com/printer_friendly/4994788*.

3. Cohen, Barney I., and Snelson, Elizabeth A. *Model Medical Staff Code of Conduct.* American Medical Association, 2008.

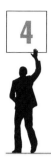

4

Just Culture Concepts: Reporting, QI, and Transparency

- Describe the importance of near-miss reporting

- Identify strategies for streamlining error reporting

Suppose you are getting confidential, anecdotal reports that over the last several months that a particular unit has been experiencing an increase in the number of incidents relating to urinary tract infections (UTI) in postoperative patients assigned to a particular staff member's unit, but there is no documented evidence to support this contention. Will any action necessarily take place if there is no data to back up what is being verbally reported?

In all likelihood, probably not, because although anecdotal data can tell a story, in order find out what it means or what we can learn from it the information needs to be collected. In order to do that, there has to be a mechanism in place as well as a nonpunitive reason for reporting when something happens that is out of the ordinary. What better way to collect such data than through an objective, systematic process? Before the Institute of Medicine's (IOM) *To Err Is Human* and the current patient safety efforts that followed, incident reporting systems were pretty much used only to report those events that had the potential for becoming a claim, or to address the error from a disciplinary perspective with those actually involved in the event, or both. But we now know that data collected from incident reporting can be a very valuable source of information. It can be used to show how and why patient safety efforts work. We have now come to realize that incident or event reporting can actually help an organization to proactively detect unsafe processes and systems, as well as identify potential patterns or trends over time. Reporting any and all events, as well as near misses and good catches, is truly a vital part of an effective and successful risk management and patient safety program.

Remember, typically senior leadership perceives its organization to have a higher rating of its patient safety culture than do the frontline staff members, who usually have a more neutral or even a negative view of the organization's current culture. And obviously, senior leadership would like to see overall survey results that are more positive in nature than negative. For example, according to the Agency for Healthcare Research and Quality's (AHRQ) *Hospital Survey on Patient Safety Culture 2008 Comparative Database Report*, which can be found on the AHRQ website, the percentage of staff members who felt that they worked on a patient-safety-focused unit was 72%. However, the percentage of staff members who still felt that their mistakes and incident reports were being held against them and/or were included in their personnel file was a whopping 44%. I find these figures amazing in light of the increased awareness by the public and the healthcare community, as well as the significant amount of education that has been conducted on patient safety since the Institute of Medicine report came out in 1999. There have been considerable efforts by the medical community to communicate internally and externally that the organization considers patient safety a priority. However, despite staff members' continued concern for themselves professionally if or when, they report an adverse event, the staff members continue to complete the surveys. I am encouraged by their willingness to still try to let leaders know about whether the culture is improving from year to year or at least from survey to survey.

Sharing Assessment Findings

Now that leadership has these data, what to do with them? First and foremost, give them to the folks who completed the survey—the staff members. The sooner you get it back to them, the sooner you can begin to solicit their ideas for solutions. More importantly, this is your "buy-in window"— that short period of time in which you, as organizational leaders, can most influence staff response.

However, be advised that this window definitely has a finite time frame before it becomes necessary to close it. This means that leadership needs to be able to communicate with staff members about the results as soon as they become available and senior managers had time to review and process them. This openness and willingness to share keeps the staff involved.

If getting the findings back out to the staff is delayed for long, staff momentum will wane, interest will be lost, and the staff will forget about it. Worse, the perception will be that leadership doesn't put this cultural change high on its priority list because it has taken so long just to share results on the survey. The staff might also feel that, at a minimum, the organization's culture and leaders do not choose to allocate the necessary resources to guide cultural change to the next level, or simply do not want to move from a punitive culture to one that is more just or fair. Simply put, staff members will most likely assume that management doesn't care enough about the frontline workers to want to change the culture and would just as soon keep the status quo.

Don't take it personally

Once results are shared, be sure to review them with a grain of salt. Rather than focusing on specific individual comments that leadership could take personally, take a look at the whole picture, focusing on patterns and trends that may be identified as needing an objective, more in-depth evaluation, or that may be of particular concern to you and your organization. Remember, this is not personal! As a perfectly normal and understandable reaction to negative comments, organizational leadership does have a tendency, at least at first blush, to be somewhat defensive. However, this approach will be an obstacle to getting the organization where it needs to be in regard to patient safety. Remember that staff members' *honest* feedback was solicited by the institution because management truly wants to know staff's perception of the current culture. Therefore, when the staff members actually do respond back as requested, they should not be penalized in any way, particularly when the information provided will be one of the many instruments that will help make the organization's case for much-needed change toward a more patient-focused culture of safety.

Positive effects of sharing data

On the other hand, knowledge can have a powerful effect, particularly at the staff level. For example, let's go back to the original scenario discussed at the beginning of the chapter to make the point: If the identified trend of an increased number of UTIs is investigated and it is discovered that all of the infections reported seem to be related to the amount of time postoperative knee replacement patients have a Foley catheter in place—and this information is shared with the orthopedic unit staff—then, between the risk manager, the appropriate department managers, and the staff, a nonpunitive approach can be taken to address the issue and prevent future infections from occurring. Changing policies, procedures, workspaces, work practices, and/or equipment—not to mention providing education, promoting the use of best and evidence-based practices, and, above all, encouraging communication—have all shown to help prevent and reduce similar events in the future.

Additionally, including staff feedback at all levels within the organization, and enhancing the work environment are both very important goals of the incident reporting process. Not only that, but staff will most likely be more inclined to report any type of event, not just the serious, potentially compensable ones, without fear of reprisals because they know that by alerting risk management whenever an unusual event occurs, they are helping to change behavior and improve the quality and safety of the care provided to the community for which the organization serves. The staff also will see the positive effect of their reporting behavior, which has a large potential to encourage further reporting. When staff aren't afraid to report those near misses, risk management can analyze the cause of those system failures and contributing factors to proactively develop action plans designed to protect patients from getting harmed in the first place.

When risk managers share the event reporting data, department managers can now see for themselves the type of events actually occurring on their units and can share that data with their staff on a regular basis, and staff can help make sure that the action plans developed to address the issues in individual departments or units have been implemented. Lastly, progress toward compliance with what was determined to be a targeted goal can be monitored and benchmarked against the other departments, as well as at the regional and national levels. Best practices can then be shared and implemented universally, with the expected outcome of improved patient safety and a reduction in patient harm.

Using Findings to Create a Plan

Survey responses also give management the information it needs as a baseline from which to start its action plan for change. This baseline will be the starting place from which future efforts can be measured for comparison as change activity starts to be implemented.

Involve staff

Once survey results are communicated back to the staff, an action plan does not have to be immediately developed and implemented. The staff's assistance in developing and putting a plan into place is critical to success. In fact, an action plan should not even be initiated without the staff's direct involvement and input. There also needs to be some concrete concept of when folks can expect that some of their suggestions or ideas will at least be considered, if not incorporated, into the final work plan. They also need to know that outcomes will be measured and that the plan's effectiveness will be evaluated.

Remember, too, that these findings actually do tell a story; some parts are good, some not so good—but, in their entirety, they do provide a snapshot of the staff's perception of the culture within the organization and just exactly what the staff has to say about that culture. Additionally, as you weed through the volumes and volumes of data that come back to you, keep in mind that these results help the board, senior leadership, medical staff, and middle management determine strategic goals and objectives for the coming years. The organization can do this by holding organizationwide "town meetings" and inviting staff members to participate or hold focus groups or inviting unit or department representatives the manager thinks would provide some, honest but objective, feedback.

Keep promises

The key is that once you have the information needed to develop a viable action plan, you must implement it and follow through! These are definitely words to live by. Leadership's credibility is on the line here and is largely dependent on whether they hold up their end of the bargain. Staff members will be very leery of words until they see some action behind them. If senior leadership says that from now on they will perform walk-arounds twice per shift and really listen to staff members while they visit each unit, the staff will expect leadership representatives to actually perform walk-arounds twice per shift. They must actually be there on their unit every day, asking questions and truly showing staff members that management really did mean what they said and is interested in the staff's feedback. If leadership doesn't show up on a regular basis as promised in the action plan, the credibility of the organization just went down the drain. Remember that when the action plan calls for some accountability on the part of leadership as well as that of the staff, it will be measured with very critical eyes.

By the same token, if leadership shows their solid commitment to changing the patient-safety culture of the organization and also shows their support of the staff's efforts to be more patient-safety-focused, the rewards will be huge. Staff members will be more likely to keep their promises to work toward a more just culture if they have witnessed the same efforts exhibited by leadership.

The Importance of Near-Miss Reporting

Although there is significant evidence that error reporting is slowly but surely becoming more important, the focus of adverse-event reporting has always been retrospective in nature. In other words, most events being evaluated are those that have already happened and have reached the patient, regardless of whether there was harm. Those events that have not yet reached the patient but continue to occur repetitively haven't, up until this point, been as important to an organization because they don't usually relate to the immediate concern of potential financial loss.

However, it is a mistake to push the near misses to the side rather than considering them to be missed opportunities. By not looking at these types of events proactively, the organization is missing out on the chance to actually find out how an event or series of similar events can be prevented. Although an organization may not want to acknowledge just how many near-miss events happen within its own four walls every day, doing so helps leadership to proactively address these missed opportunities to improve performance, promote patient safety, and prevent patient harm. Institutions willing to embrace this approach begin to understand that the ultimate goal of high-quality patient care provided in a professional and caring manner should at every level outweigh any remaining misgivings about reporting any type of adverse event, bad outcome, or near miss/missed opportunities.

Additionally, institutions not only begin to realize that the event could possibly have been prevented, but they learn how to objectively delve deeper into the reasons a near-miss event occurred in the first place. A successful action plan can be developed that will most likely, if not absolutely, help the organization better understand the levels of risk involved when at-risk behavior continues.

Sentinel Events and Root Cause Analysis

Another important reason the reporting of medical errors is so imperative to a healthcare organization is that The Joint Commission has patient safety and performance improvement standards specifically relating to requirements for managing the follow-up of serious adverse outcomes, otherwise known as sentinel events. The Joint Commission's definition of a sentinel event is:

...an unexpected occurrence involving death or serious physical or psychological injury, or the risk thereof. Serious injury specifically includes loss of limb or function. The phrase 'or the risk thereof' includes any process variation for which a recurrence would carry a significant chance of a serious adverse outcome. Such events are called 'sentinel' because they signal the need for immediate investigation and response.[1]

Further, all Joint Commission–accredited organizations are expected to identify and respond appropriately to all sentinel events; the most commonly performed response is what is known as a root cause analysis (RCA), which The Joint Commission defines as "a process for identifying the basic or causal factors that underlie variation in performance, including the occurrence or possible occurrence of a sentinel event."[2] In other words, after convening a multidisciplinary team of providers and/or other ancillary department staff members, an RCA should be established to focus on process problems, not people problems, and should utilize those generally accepted standardized tools developed to assist organizations with identifying potential opportunities for improvements in processes or systems that would, in time, prevent similar events from occurring in the future.

What the RCA also forces is the continuing question of "Why?" until it just can't be asked or answered anymore. The Joint Commission requires that an action plan be completed within 45 days of the date it was determined that a sentinel event occurred. This plan must address not only those action items relating to the specific event, but also must incorporate those action items developed to address the prevention of similar events in the future. In addition, it should address individual responsibilities for specific action items, timelines, and how monitoring and evaluating for effectiveness will be handled.

Failure Modes and Effects Analysis

Whereas an RCA addresses actions taken following the occurrence of a sentinel event, and is reactive in nature, failure modes and effects analysis (FMEA) takes on the proactive approach of identifying and mitigating those potential hazards that can cause patient harm before they have a chance to occur.

This activity is also a Joint Commission requirement, with at least one FMEA to be conducted annually on a "high-risk process," which can be identified through various reporting mechanisms and is based in part on what The Joint Commission has identified as being high-risk issues and on what the hospital itself has identified as being a potential issue that needs to be addressed.

The FMEA team should be multidisciplinary in nature, ultimately taking about one year to fully complete and implement. The FMEA is where the reporting of those near misses becomes so important: If a pattern or trend is identified through the reporting of these types of events that could and probably will cause harm but haven't yet, the organization has a golden opportunity to proactively prevent the events from occurring. What better way to find out about potential hazardous conditions than through the organization's event reporting system?

Now that it is understood why the voluntary internal reporting of any type of potentially serious event is so important, how can organizations not only encourage reporting, but also make it easier for the staff to do so?

Streamlining the Error Reporting Process

Error reporting can be difficult, and staff may fear reporting or believe they are too busy to report. It is critical to make the error reporting process as easy as possible and to make it worthwhile for staff members and the hospital system as a whole. Staff members must see how reporting can help the hospital, help the patients, and, sometimes, help them as human beings who have made a mistake. Certain steps should be taken to ensure reporting happens easily and often.

 Creating a Just Culture

Give a reason

First, educate the staff about why incidents should be reported, particularly addressing the difference between serious events with possible bad outcomes and near misses—those events that never reach the patient, either through sheer luck or by staff intervention, and that do not results in patient harm. However, a near miss indicates that the potential for injury existed and, even if the outcome was okay that time, a similar event might happen again in the future with negative outcomes. If we look at the processes associated with the event now, before it happens again, we can anticipate being able to completely prevent it from happening in the future.

Additionally, emphasis must be made on reassuring the staff that incident reports are maintained in the utmost confidential manner and that every effort will be made to protect the report from being disclosed unnecessarily or inappropriately. The staff members need to know and rely on the organization's position of a nonpunitive reporting process and feel that leadership view incident event reporting as an opportunity to alert risk management about an adverse event so steps can be taken toward appropriate action, if necessary.

More importantly, however, the staff need to know that whether an actual event or near miss has occurred, appropriate action steps have been or will be taken to address the issue and that these are always lesson-learning opportunities. This attitude conveys that the event was "significant enough to have had an impact on organization operations, was factually correct, identified a specific process or decision that reduces or eliminates the potential for failures or mishaps, or reinforces a positive result."[3]

Return the favor

Just as much as the hospital needs to know of adverse events, the staff needs to know outcomes of the patients who suffered them. If an adverse event has occurred, and the patient ends up being transferred to another floor or another facility, staff members want to know how the patient is doing. The manager's responsibility is to provide that feedback to them. For most healthcare clinicians, making a mistake is very difficult to handle internally. When errors happen and clinicians "fess up," the initial response is to want to fix it and make the patient healthy immediately. Clinicians are often hardest on themselves, expecting more of themselves than what would ordinarily be considered reasonable by other clinicians in the same or a similar set of circumstances. For that reason, closure is very important to staff members. It allows staff members to decompress and to stop beating themselves up. It lets them see that in most cases, the patient is not seriously harmed and will be fine. Even if the patient does not have a good outcome, at least the employee is aware and can be mentored through this learning process to ensure that a similar event won't be repeated.

Make it easy

Organizations need to make incident reporting much more user-friendly, and the reporting process should include clearly understood instructions for how a report is to be completed and what information should be contained in it. For example, the IOM recommends a combination of objective data entry with a section for narrative information, including:

- The discovery—who and how it was discovered

- The event—type of near miss/adverse event

- Where, when, and who was involved

- Severity and preventability of the event—likelihood of recurrence

- Ancillary information—patient and product information, as applicable

- Detailed analysis[4]

One of the most common complaints organizations hear from their staff about the event reporting process is that it is difficult and tedious to complete (e.g., locating the hardcopy report form and taking the time to fill it out). Additionally, although staff members are encouraged to complete the form as soon as possible after the event has occurred, while the memory of all of the circumstances surrounding the event is fresh and can be clearly documented, sometimes it is just not possible for them to do so until after the shift is over. Before a formalized reporting process is put into place, it is always a good idea to solicit staff's input as to what the common barriers are to incident reporting. Leadership should be prepared to address the following:

- Assuring staff that they will be provided feedback on any actions taken after an event has been reported

- Assuring staff that the incident reporting process developed and implemented will be easy to access and use, as well as efficient, and thereby will take a minimal amount of time to complete

- Assuring staff that incident reporting is not punitive and is only a mechanism by which a deviation from the norm is being communicated to the appropriate individuals

- Including common taxonomy that clearly defines what should be reported

- Educating physicians and other healthcare providers regarding the purpose of an incident reporting system so that there is a clear understanding of how reporting events can help improve patient safety at all levels of care

- Assuring staff that reports can be submitted anonymously if preferred

- Educating about both actual and potential harm, so that it is understood that evaluation of process is just as important as investigation of an event

- Educating staff about how reporting and investigating an incident assists risk management with management of the defense strategy of the claim, should a lawsuit be filed

- Assuring staff of the ease by which an event can be reported, including minimal time required to complete the report—because it is understood that patient care is top priority

If the process is difficult for staff members to navigate, the incident report won't be completed and an opportunity to learn from mistakes is missed. Systems for reporting events should be simple and easy for the user to access. The "keep it simple, stupid," or "KISS," principle particularly applies with respect to ease of staff reporting adverse events. More and more vendors have developed online, Web-based adverse-event reporting systems that are user-friendly, are easily accessible, have only minimal required fields, and take no more than a few minutes to complete.

Additionally, these systems can generate reports to show possible patterns and trends, drill down to specific details, and put the onus back on the department manager in regard to ownership of the process. Managers are responsible for all actions and interactions on their units, especially when it comes to the types of events being reported by their staff. If immediate access to data can be made available to the manager, that data can be reviewed, possible patterns and/or trends can be identified, and managers can begin to engage the staff in coming up with patient safety solutions based on the types of incidents occurring on their own units. This way, staff are involved, better solutions that work to prevent harm and that can be shared with others are developed, and similar events won't be repeated in other areas/departments of the hospital.

To encourage event reporting, organizations should be urged to keep the event reporting process as simple and as easy to use as possible and to explore electronic alternatives to paper event reporting. Studies have shown that as error reporting improves and error-detection rates increase, the severity of the errors eventually decreases. There also seems to be a tremendous reduction in the number of serious adverse events reported when an organization has created a patient safety culture that positively reinforces safe behaviors and a disciplinary system that allows employees to come forward and report their mistakes without fear of reprisals. In his *Just Culture Primer*, David Marx sums it up by saying, "Not reporting the error, preventing the system and others from learning … is the greatest evil of all."[5]

Disclosure to Patients/Families

There is one final, although clearly important, aspect of event reporting that absolutely cannot be left out of the equation: when and what to tell patients/families whenever a medical error has taken place. I have found this to be one of the most, if not *the* most, challenging aspects of a quality, risk, and/or patient safety professional's job: To balance the needs of the patient with those of the organization, as well as those of the healthcare provider involved in the event. What needs to be emphasized here is that a collaborative process that has been proven to promote a mutual trust between all involved—ensuring that events will be handled appropriately, honestly, and objectively—will make the difficult task of communicating with the family about the event a bit easier. Such a process also sends a clear message to patients and their families that everyone involved in the event is working together toward ensuring that their need for an open discussion will be met. Patients and families should understand that their questions can be asked and then answered by those most knowledgeable about the circumstances. This approach also sends a message to staff and healthcare providers that their work environment promotes a just culture—a culture that, in turn, leads to staff believing that reporting and disclosing about an event is the right thing to do for the sake of the patient and future patients, and leads to a more conducive opportunity to learn from mistakes made.

From the patient's perspective, of course he or she wants to know whenever an error in his or her care has taken place, particularly when continued patient safety efforts are today's current focus and with communication now viewed as being a key factor in preventing adverse events and patient harm. In general, the public feels that healthcare clinicians should not only feel an obligation to disclose the error but should also exhibit a willingness to discuss any and all circumstances surrounding the error and be prepared to answer any questions the patient and/or family may have during this process. It is, after all, the patient's body, and he or she has a right to know about anything that may have happened to it, as well as to make any decisions regarding further care. Additionally, it is not unusual for the patient/family and the public to believe that it is the clinician's duty to the patient, to him or herself, to the organization, and to the medical profession to tell the truth about what happened.

Although a healthcare clinician often agrees that it is the right thing to do to disclose to a patient whenever there has been a medical error relating to the patient's care, there is a real and distinct fear that once the patient learns of the error, a medical malpractice lawsuit will follow, putting the clinician in a no-win situation, at least in his or her mind. Although data are not clear about whether patients are more likely to file a lawsuit once disclosure of an error has been acknowledged, in many cases, when asked, patients/families indicated that although the extent of the harm was the true determining factor for whether a claim was filed, in most cases, they filed a lawsuit as a last resort for obtaining information they felt had been purposefully withheld from them and not necessarily because a clinician had made a mistake. In other words, the patient's perception that the physician was not completely honest may not be the direct reason for filing a lawsuit, but it certainly can be an underlying contributory factor for doing so. This same patient often feels that clinicians held back when discussing the circumstances surrounding the event or that there was no accompanying apology expressing regret that the event occurred.

In most cases, patients do not distinguish the difference between an apology reflecting regret that an event occurred without admitting responsibility and an apology made by the provider who actually caused harm. It is the perception that the provider showed sincerity and empathy with the patient/family that is the more important concern. In fact, studies also show that only about 3%–5% of patients harmed from negligent medical care actually file a claim or lawsuit.[6] When enacting disclosure policies that remove any negative consequences, there is early anecdotal evidence that legal fees and other associated expenses can be reduced by as much as 50%.

Supporting Staff

As indicated previously, the patient and family are not the only ones affected by a medical error that resulted in an adverse outcome. Clinicians, for the most part, are what I would typically consider being "type A" personalities and often have such high expectations of themselves that they tend to be greatly affected when it comes to making a medical error; as a result, there can an enormous amount of emotional distress experienced by the provider responsible for committing the error. There is very little training available to providers about how to deal with these sensitive kinds of circumstances. At the same time, the organization could have a very difficult and somewhat volatile situation on its hands if the disclosure is not managed appropriately, and may be under strain as well. Here are a few tips for providers when disclosing information about medical errors to patients:

- Ensure that the organization has a disclosure process in place that takes into consideration the sensitivity of each situation and of all parties involved.

- Ask for assistance from the organization's risk managers and turn to colleagues for support. Determine who will be the primary communicator in advance, while allowing for others involved to add to the discussion when asked or when it is felt necessary.

- Plan for and practice how best to communicate with the patient/family about the event; the more prepared the communicator is, the less likely the chance for any misunderstanding or miscommunication that could lead to an unpleasant patient/family response.

- Objectively review the facts of the event before the meeting takes place and focus on those during the discussion.

- Find an appropriate venue that is comfortable and private.

Creating a Just Culture

- Keep attendees to only those most appropriate to be there and make sure the facilitator is experienced in the disclosure process.

- Be aware of the influence that body language and nonverbal cues can have on how disclosure is perceived by others involved in the discussion.

- Be considerate of the fact that culture of the patient/family, their ethnicity, socioeconomic background, and religion, can influence how they perceive the healthcare environment.

- Get a feel for what the patient already knows.

- Use language that is simple and easy for the patient and the family to understand, and speak slowly when providing basic information to the patient and/or family about the event as soon as is reasonably possible. Promptly follow up with additional information as soon it becomes available.

- Keep the conversation interactive by frequently encouraging the patient/family to ask questions or make comments.

- Apologize and express sincere regret that the event occurred but don't acknowledge responsibility until that outcome has truly been determined.

- Plan to maintain follow-up communication with the patient/family on a regular basis and include information about action plan progress.

- Offer support and referrals as needed to the patient, family, and the providers of care.

Demonstrating a Just Culture

Organizations truly living a just culture promote communication between caregivers at all levels, ensure event reporting through positively reinforcing that the information received will help to evaluate current systems and make improvements when concerns are identified, and demonstrate to patients and families that transparency throughout the system is the norm. These organizations are true leaders in the efforts toward promoting patient safety and preventing patient harm. They use the information obtained through incident reporting to set strategic patient safety goals. By putting patient safety first, and providing for the allocation of necessary resources, such as manpower or technology that will assist risk managers and patient safety officers as they strive for patient care excellence, they are sending a message to their communities that patient safety is a priority initiative. Although it may seem that this movement toward a more patient-centered culture is slow in catching on within the healthcare industry, it is beginning to take hold, if only one step, and one hospital, at a time.

References

1. The Joint Commission, *www.jointcommission.org*.

2. Ibid.

3. *Data for Safety: Turning Lessons Learned into Actionable Knowledge*. American Society for Healthcare Risk Management of the American Hospital Association, 2008.

4. Aspden, P., Corrigan, J.M., Wolcott, J., and Erickson, S.M. *Patient Safety: Standard of Care*. National Academies Press, 2004.

5. Marx, David. *Patient Safety and the "Just Culture": A Primer for Health Care Executives*. Trustees of Columbia University, 2001: 27.

6. Gallagher, Thomas H., Studdert, David, and Levinson, Wendy. "Disclosing harmful medical errors to patients," *New England Journal of Medicine* 356 (2007): 2713–2719.

 Creating a Just Culture

Implementation Strategies

- Name implementation steps to a just and safe culture

- Identify positive tactics for supporting a safe and just culture

Up to this point, the groundwork has been laid for your organization to conceptually accept moving toward a just culture. Now the question is, what strategies are needed to actually implement this change and how does an organization begin?

First and foremost, it goes without saying that we all want to do the right thing, at the right time, for the right patient the first time, and every time thereafter, without making a mistake or causing harm, ever. And in a perfect world, that's what would always happen—we would take good care of our patients, who in turn would always have great outcomes. Unfortunately, it's not a perfect world and, at least in my book, the one sure thing in this life is that every healthcare provider will make at least one error during the course of his or her career. Whether it will ever actually reach the patient is irrelevant. The fact is, an error will still be made, which results in at least one of the following outcomes:

- Actual event, with patient harm

- Actual event, with no patient harm

- Near miss, with no patient harm, but that had the potential to cause harm

We also know now that the majority of errors occur from systems failures or process problems, and we know that if we focus on and fix the process, we will have more success in achieving safer patient care conditions than if we target people problems or punish providers for making those errors. It is already well known that how an organization manages its event reporting system tells a lot about the organization's culture. It only follows that an organization with a robust event reporting database in all likelihood has a positive culture of patient safety in which staff members are very comfortable reporting, knowing that there won't be punitive action taken against them. However, we do not discount accountability when an error is made, particularly in light of our understanding of the set of algorithms that help us determine whether the behavior was human error only (i.e., those thoughtless mistakes we make every day, such as clicking on the wrong diet choice for a patient), at-risk behavior (e.g., being interrupted and inadvertently bringing the wrong medicine to the wrong patient), or reckless behavior (e.g., a physician's order for pain medication is disregarded because staff members have determined the patient to be drug-seeking, and shortly thereafter, the patient's condition deteriorates). We also know that those who have instituted a culture of patient safety seem to have followed several strategies to ensure successful implementation.

The Dana-Farber Cancer Institute, in conjunction with the American Hospital Association, has published a free and terrific checklist tool entitled "Strategies for Leadership Hospital Executives and Their Role in Patient Safety," which was designed to assist leaders in determining where their organizations are along their journey toward a just culture. For those organizations wanting to make the change, the following are some steps that can be taken as they begin their transition toward a more just and fair culture. For a sample timeline of steps toward implementing a just culture, see Figure 5.1.

Implementation Steps

A healthcare organization's staff members, from leadership to frontline staff, have to understand the concept of just culture, agree with the principles, and practice it every day. However, to ensure a hospital is operated 100% in a just culture manner, there are steps to take at the beginning of your journey. A healthcare organization would also be wise to review these steps occasionally and ensure everything is being done to support a just culture.

FIGURE
5.1

Just culture implementation timeline sample

The following is a timeline based on collaborative model.

Task	Responsible Party	Participants	Completion Date
Initial just culture training, to be held at ABC Hospital	1. Outside consultant to teach 2. Senior leadership representative to coordinate	Senior leadership; quality, risk, and patient safety managers; managers from Pharmacy, HR, Occupational Health, Patient Care Services	March 2011
Recruit other area hospitals to establish a collaborative that implement a just culture, and working with outside consultants, work together toward common implementation date	1. Outside consultant to assist with recruiting 2. Senior leadership representative to coordinate appts with other interested hospitals	Leadership representatives from other hospitals, outside consultants	August 31, 2011
1. Interdisciplinary team formed composed of representatives from all collaborative hospitals; consider inclusion of State Hospital Association and/ or State Patient Safety Organization 2. Additional training for collaborative hospital members	1. Senior leadership representative from each collaborative hospital to appoint team members and report to ABC Hospital designee 2. If participating, State Hospital Assn and PSO to formally notify ABC Hospital designee of agreement 3. Outside consultant to conduct additional training	As determined by each collaborative hospital, State Hospital Association and PSO	October 31, 2011
Monthly phone call meetings for consultation and sharing of processes used for training, implementation, and future planning	ABC Hospital designee to coordinate calls	1. Outside consultant 2. State Hospital Assn designee 3. PSO designee	December 1, 2011– December 31, 2013

| FIGURE 5.1 | Just culture implementation timeline sample (cont.) | | |

Task	Responsible Party	Participants	Completion Date
1. Leadership training on a "Learning, Just and Accountable Culture –" two-hour orientation and overview 2. Include introduction of just culture algorithm used to deal with review of incidents and for situations involving disciplinary action	Outside consultant	Leadership designees from each of the collaborative hospitals, state hospital association, and patient safety organization (PSO)	February 28, 2011
Completion of online just culture training modules on outside consultant website	Outside consultant to maintain documentation of participants completing modules	Leadership designees from each of the collaborative hospitals, state hospital association, and PSO	April 30, 2011
Incident report form to be revised to include just culture principles	Designees from each of the collaborative hospitals	Representatives from each collaborative hospital's Quality, Risk, Patient Safety, Patient Care Services, and ancillary departments	August 31, 2011
Continue to meet to plan means of moving just culture principles into organizational policies and procedures as appropriate	Designees from each of the collaborative hospitals	Leadership designees from each of the collaborative hospitals, state hospital association, and PSO	September 1, 2011–April 30, 2012
1. Just culture topic included at monthly department head/leadership meetings (review of some component of just culture principles 2. Just culture newsletter sent out to leadership as new editions are published	Team members from each of the collaborative hospitals	Leadership team/department heads at each collaborative hospital	October 2011–Ongoing

 Creating a Just Culture

FIGURE
5.1

Just culture implementation timeline sample (cont.)

Task	Responsible Party	Participants	Completion Date
1. Procedure for training new leaders developed and implemented 2. All new organizational leaders to receive just culture training at leadership orientation	Designees from each of the collaborative hospitals	All newly hired leaders/ department heads	February 28, 2012
1. Just culture principles discussed with each Medical Executive Committee, and peer review process use of the principles reviewed	Senior leadership designees	All Medical Staff leaders	August 31, 2012
2. Just culture principles included in new employee handbook for distribution to new employees 3. "Just Culture" principles included in revised employee standards of behavior	Team members from each of the collaborative hospitals	Leadership designees from each of the collaborative hospitals, state hospital association, and PSO	
4. Participate on work group with state hospital association, PSO, state licensing boards, and departments of health to incorporate principles into their investigation and disciplinary review processes	Team members from each of the collaborative hospitals	Leadership designees from each of the collaborative hospitals, state hospital association, and PSO, along with representatives of state officials	

FIGURE 5.1 **Just culture implementation timeline sample (cont.)**

Task	Responsible Party	Participants	Completion Date
1. Reinforce just culture principles at quarterly Medical Staff meetings, with explanation that principles are now included in formal peer review process 2. Root cause analysis process under review for revision to include just culture principles and change form to include the "three behaviors"	Leadership designees from each of the collaborative hospitals, state hospital association, and PSO	All Medical Staff members Team members from each of the collaborative hospitals	November 30, 2012
New leader orientation process changed and implemented, also now part of HR's New Leader training process, using outside consultant's materials and online training resource	1. Outside consultant 2. Team members from each of the collaborative hospitals 3. Leadership designees from each of the collaborative hospitals, state hospital association, and PSO	New orientees	January 1, 2013

Adapted from the Minnesota Hospital Association, www.mnhospitals.org.

Step 1: Leadership buy-in

If the culture of the organization is to truly be patient-safety-focused, then it is absolutely critical that leadership set the example by communicating to all employees, including managers, medical staff, and board members, that patient safety is a priority organizational strategic goal. There are many steps leadership can take to ensure that they mean business when they say patient safety is an

 Creating a Just Culture

important component of success for the organization. The following is a checklist for leadership to ensure they are communicating this priority effectively:

- Make sure patient safety issues are discussed at senior leadership and board meetings.

- Do walk-arounds and talk to staff about what they perceive are serious patient safety issues.

- Ensure senior leadership representatives are involved in performance improvement, and patient safety and risk management committees; their attendance and participation should be required.

- Ensure patient safety education is presented at new-staff and medical staff orientation programs, as well as at regularly scheduled educational sessions.

- Provide a "Lessons Learned" forum where staff can present actual adverse events to their colleagues and ask them to provide to the group their plans for how these issues will be prevented from happening again.

- If a plan was successful, ask staff to share how this was accomplished with the rest of the organization and promote these successes throughout the organization.

- Make patient safety a part of the competencies and performance evaluations for every hospital employee, the medical staff, and the governing board.

Step 2: Formation of a patient safety culture committee

Form a patient safety culture committee, task force, or initiative composed of representatives from nursing, ancillary clinical and nonclinical departments, middle and senior leadership, and the medical staff. This team of committed individuals will eventually serve as just culture champions for the entire organization, as well as a resource for assistance and guidance to support the staff's efforts. Members of this group will also be crucial in helping to build an awareness of what the staff, as well as leadership, perceives the current culture to be and will serve as cheerleaders during the patient safety culture assessment survey process, encouraging survey completion housewide. As discussed previously, this step has probably already been completed. Also as discussed previously, the results are usually an initial surprise to leadership, because their perception of the current culture will most likely differ from that of the frontline staff.

Step 3: Assessing current culture

If it hasn't been done by now, then it is time to assess the organization's current culture of patient safety. As discussed previously, the Agency for Healthcare Research and Quality's Culture of Patient Safety Survey is an excellent tool (although there are others) to determine the initial baseline opinions of the survey takers with respect to the organization's current culture. The best practice is to resurvey every six months, focusing on those areas most needing immediate improvement, until measurement determines that the organization has at least met its minimum target for improvement. Once improvements are identified as being more stable with respect to the rate of progress, then the survey should be conducted every year.

Step 4: Education

The next step is to educate senior leadership, members of the board, and other key operations managers about the just culture movement by conducting a formal just culture workshop or other full-day session. It is at this point that an outside expert on the subject would be the most credible instructor, someone like David Marx or James Reason, who can truly do justice to the topic and who can motivate the attendees into action. It has been my experience that, in many environments, educational sessions conducted by outside experts have a more lasting effect than those provided by in-house staff members, regardless of credentials. Inviting someone outside of the hospital to speak also validates the message that the hospital's patient safety staff has been trying to communicate, usually for a long time prior to bringing an expert in to conduct the session.

Next, develop an orientation training program on patient safety and just culture for all new directors, managers, and supervisors coming on board, as well as for those who have been with the organization for some time. Include the topic of accountability as part of the program and encourage participants to work with human resources prior to utilizing a disciplinary process or taking any action. Develop a similar program to be presented annually as a reminder of the organization's commitment to fairness and accountability.

In most cases, once senior leadership and managers have been brought on board, formal educational sessions for the staff may not be necessary, depending on how comfortable mid-level managers feel about communicating to their staff what they have learned and ways in which patient safety can be improved. In fact, in many instances, educating the rest of the staff can really be incorporated into the routine and practical operations of the institution. However, if the organization feels that formal staff training is necessary, there is no need to start from scratch. There are several programs already out there online that can be adapted to meet the organization's needs. For more information, *www.justculture.org* is a great place to start looking into how education can be provided.

Step 5: Policy, procedure, and protocol development

Revise policies, procedures, and protocols (particularly those policies relating to expectations for behavior) and continue efforts through routine orientation, during routinely scheduled competency training, and at unit-specific education programs whenever possible. Any policies that do not promote a just culture should be eliminated, specifically those relating to punishment for errors. Policies that will need to be revised include your incident reporting policy, sentinel event policy, disclosure policy, patient complaint/grievance process, job descriptions, codes of conduct, medical staff bylaws, rules and regulations, and the like.

Any document that addresses the consequences for behavior and the management of adverse events will need to be revised to reconcile professional accountability and the need to create a safe environment to report medical errors. In other words, the staff need to know that if an event occurred because of a system failure or flaw, then the organization accepts responsibility and accountability, and the individual will not be punished for something that was out of his or her control.

Leadership will need to understand that the reasons for clinical outcomes and events should not be the focus, nor should those involved be prejudged. Any rush to blame individuals is to be avoided. Rather, there should be an attempt to understand at the time the event occurred the circumstances and context for the actions and decision-making. The main focus of this analysis is on system failures—with any and all subsequent analyses and proceedings conducted with fairness, within the legislative and legal frameworks, and in accordance with established hospital policy and/or bylaws. The rights of all individuals are protected, for both employees and patients, and policies and procedures should reflect language that addresses:

- Leadership's commitment to and support of the purpose of quality improvement

- Leadership appropriately protecting any and all quality improvement information from legal, regulatory, or other proceedings

- The organization's intolerance of intentionally unsafe actions, reckless actions, disregard for the welfare of patients or staff, or other willful misconduct and misbehavior

Defining unacceptable behavior

There is "a collective understanding of where the line should be drawn between blameless and blameworthy actions."[1] For this stage of implementation, it is vital that representatives from human resources be included on the team established for policy review to ensure that the management of the staff based on a just culture complies with state and federal statutes. The differences between the types of behaviors that are acceptable (i.e., making an error through a simple mistake) versus behaviors that are unacceptable and considered to be reckless in nature need to be clearly defined and identified. Keep in mind that implementing a just culture should be a continuous performance improvement process and, as human errors and at-risk and reckless behaviors are identified, how and why these errors occurred needs to be investigated and evaluated and, when necessary, new processes need to be put into place that are designed to prevent the error from happening in the first place.

Staff members also need to know the difference between what is human error versus what is at-risk or reckless behavior, with a clear understanding that there are consequences associated with the two unacceptable types of behavior. The steps addressing the appropriate disciplinary action should be included in the new or revised policies. Examples of what would constitute acceptable versus unacceptable behavior are noted in Figure 5.2:

FIGURE 5.2 — **Three types of behavior**

	Type	Definition	Example	Action to be taken
Acceptable	Human error	Inadvertent action	Leaving sugar out of a recipe; accidental delay in administering medication	Change to processes, procedure, training, or design
Unacceptable	At-risk behavior	Unintentional risk-taking	Driving 5–10 miles over the speed limit on a limited access highway (standard work-around); answering cell phone in the OR (against policy); failing to review patient record diligently, so misses patient allergy to penicillin, and administers	Remove incentives for work-arounds and at-risk behavior; create incentives for following policies; increase situational awareness
	Reckless behavior	Intentional risk-taking	Driving 95 miles per hour where the speed limit is 65; working under the influence of alcohol or illegal drugs	Remedial or punitive action

 Creating a Just Culture

The medical staff is not immune, nor should it be excluded from policies or procedures or their implementation. In fact, it is essential that medical staff be included in this process, particularly in hospitals with a community model of the medical staff, meaning members are not employed but are privileged to care for their patients in healthcare organizations of all settings, and therefore healthcare providers need to understand that similar concepts apply to them as well.

For example:

Dr. Smith has scheduled a patient for surgery. She has followed proper preoperative procedures for checking to make sure she has the right patient going to the operating room for the correct procedure but fails to notice the red allergy sticker on the chart indicating that the patient is allergic to penicillin and administers it prophylactically to prevent the potential for infection before the start of the procedure. The patient immediately develops difficulty breathing, and emergency measures are required to stabilize the patient before the surgery is initiated.

This would be considered a human error, and the physician would be reminded to check the chart for allergies before administering any medications. However, even though the error was made by the physician, which would make this type of event fall under the human error category, during a discussion with the physician and the staff afterward, it is also suggested that there should be some trigger tools that would help providers remember to follow certain guidelines with respect to checking for possible allergies. For example, to improve the notification process, use a sticker designed with larger letters or place a red wristband on the patient that says **ALLERGY** in big, bold letters. Both tactics might help prevent a similar occurrence from happening in the future.

Let's consider another case:

Dr. Triver's patient is in the operating room and he is about to start the procedure when his cell phone rings and he answers it, even though there is a well-known policy that requires all cell phones to be turned off during an operative procedure. Dr. Triver has the right patient for the correct procedure, but because he is on the phone, he has not reviewed the chart or seen the sticker indicating the patient's penicillin allergy and he administers it. The patient develops difficulty breathing. and emergency measures are necessary to stabilize him.

By definition, this is reckless behavior, and as such, appropriate steps to address this behavior might include contacting the chief of surgery and the risk management and patient safety staff, arranging for a meeting with the surgeon as quickly as possible after the event, and discussing with the surgeon that his actions were exactly the reason why the policy was developed. He was made aware of the policy at a previous medical staff meeting, and his deliberate violation of the policy requires some sort of disciplinary action and documentation in his credentialing file that will be considered at the time of reappointment.

Step 6: Sustain the gain

Now that just culture has been embraced by leadership and is being incorporated into practices, policies, and procedures, strategies are still necessary to maintain the progress made and encourage it to continue throughout the organization. Among them are:

- **Routine walk-arounds by senior leadership.** Staff members need to see that leadership is easily accessible to discuss any concerns and is not sitting in an "ivory tower," out of touch with what the staff are dealing with on a daily basis. This is also an opportunity for leadership to see for itself some of the situations the staff face every day.

- **Ensuring that staffing is adequate to meet the safety needs of the organization's patients.** Although organizations must constantly deal with maintaining a balanced financial picture, staff members also need to be reassured that patient safety will not be compromised and that leadership will support maintaining adequate staffing resources to meet, and even exceed, patient needs.

- **Reinforcing the need to report near misses or good catches in addition to the actual adverse events.** Staff members should be encouraged to continue reporting events, no matter if they initially perceive the event to be serious or insignificant. Managers can support this endeavor by providing routine feedback to staff members on a monthly basis about the types of events being reported and any follow-up actions that may have been necessary to resolve issues. This is an important factor for staff members, because many times after they report an event, they would like to know the outcome of any investigation but they don't feel comfortable asking about how the issue was addressed. If staff members are involved in a root cause analysis (RCA), encourage them to share what they learned with their peers, management, and the medical staff so that similar events can be prevented in the future. Reassure staff members that just because an error is reported internally to the appropriate individuals for the necessary action and follow-up, it does not mean it will be accessible to the plaintiff's counsel should a lawsuit be filed as a result of the error.

Note: Although most states do not have statutes providing complete incident report protection from discovery, a few do, and Maryland is one of them. However, with the New Patient Safety Act of 2005, incidents reported through a designated patient safety organization are protected from discovery. Still, there are some practices that will maximize any protections afforded, such as refraining from making copies of reports, keeping them maintained in the office of risk management, and noting on each report that it is being reviewed under the auspices of quality improvement and/or as work produced under attorney-client privilege. Reports should be maintained confidentially and should not be discussed inappropriately or outside the proper venue.

- **Continuing teamwork training on a routine basis.** When staff members work as a team toward the common goal of promoting patient safety and preventing patient harm and see the successful outcomes, even the small ones, staff members will begin to see that they can succeed on other patient safety projects as well. They should know that the process outcomes are not flukes but are organized approaches resulting in a higher rate of success than unorganized, unfocused ones.

- **Sustained peer support and understanding.** Each staff member must know that he or she can count on each other for support, guidance, and the reassurance that every effort has been made to provide the safest quality care possible. Not only that, but team members working in different departments will get a new appreciation of what other departments do, what they do for patient care, how they interrelate with each other, and how they can help each other better coordinate patient care. And as time goes by, team members begin to trust each other more to do the right thing.

- **Tying it all together.** Staff members will also begin to see the correlation between the hospital's patient safety projects and other hospital quality or risk management initiatives, such as the Joint Commission survey process, any statewide or regional work groups or initiatives, compliance activities for other accrediting bodies, etc. Additionally, by sharing information about reported events, both unit-specific and organizationwide, staff members will be able to identify possible patterns and trends and can make relevant contributions to a more potentially successful action plan developed to address the specific trend proactively, before patient harm can occur.

- **Redistributing a culture of patient safety assessment every year to all employees.** Explain that with staff assistance, leadership will be able to determine progress by comparing what the culture was like at baseline with what it is now. Explain that staff too will be able to see how far the organization has come each year, and in what areas they have improved, as well as in what areas improvements still need to be made. It is important for staff members to know how far they have come and how their efforts have shaped the improvements made in their organization's patient safety initiatives. It is just as important for them to see that leadership relies on the staff to continue to effect positive change and move toward a more patient-safety-focused environment.

Barriers and Challenges to Implementation

Of course, there will be challenges to implementing a more patient-safety and just-culture-focused approach to providing care. Some barriers to consider are:

- **Lack of structure.** Signs of a lack of structure would be meetings that are not regularly scheduled or spotty attendance by the assigned members. It is imperative that the members of the team understand the expectations, goals, and objectives of the group. Explain what the goal expectations are and why they were established, who will be responsible for what tasks, and provide an initial timeline for completing specific actions necessary for success. This timeline should be somewhat flexible with respect to when certain tasks can be reasonably completed, but the final date of project implementation should be an absolute deadline that is not to be changed or extended without good reason. This assures senior leadership of the team's commitment to accomplishing the goals it has set forth, and it also reassures the team that this will not be a futile effort; their roles play an important part in ensuring that the organization is committed to a fair patient safety culture.

- **The continued existence of silos.** Evidence of working in silos—or working in an environment that keeps departments and units separate and lacks cohesiveness—includes a lack of collaboration among members of the just culture team, each failing to consider getting outside their own comfort zone and failing to consider how an event affects more than one department or unit. Make sure each team member understands that when an error occurs, in most instances, the process usually affects more than one department or unit, which can, and usually does, have a domino effect on the whole organization. Once staff understand the role that other departments/units have in the current process, members can then build new processes while keeping the function of others in mind. This builds a sense of teamwork and creates processes that are better suited for practical application.

- **Personality issues.** There is always some potential for conflict between individuals that has to be addressed and put aside to ensure that patient safety is the primary focus. Keep emotion out of the mix whenever possible by addressing potential personality conflicts with the individuals involved prior to the initial team meeting. Emphasize that individuals were chosen to be members of the team because their unique insight is crucial to the success of the team's charge. Acknowledge your understanding of each individual's perspective, but stress the importance of leaving personal feelings behind. Reiterate that the focus needs to be on improving processes that move the organization toward a more patient-centered culture.

- **Manager resistance.** For whatever reason, the manager may not be completely on board, and may be skeptical as to whether the team's work will be worth the effort. Again, highlight that without leadership buy-in, any efforts made will be pointless. Explain that the management's active and supportive participation will set an example for the rest of the team.

And, in addition to the potential barriers, there are also some potential challenges to consider:

- **Managers must be adequately trained to effectively conduct event investigations and follow-up.** Require managers to attend training sessions on how to thoroughly complete an investigation of an event, including knowledge of what steps are involved and how follow-up is expected to be completed. This may include advising staff of the outcome of your investigation, and explaining how they can be actively involved in the follow-up process

- **Staff must get past the human error approach in order to address the potentially broken process.** Though clearly a person who commits an error should be held accountable, staff need to know that this will be appropriately addressed. However, emphasize that the main goal is to focus on how the process leading up to the error could be improved to ensure that a similar event does not occur. Involve these individuals as members of the team to help design a better process.

- **There must be a focus on future prevention.** Although everyone on the team will be understandably affected by a severe event outcome, remind staff that developing a solution will help to prevent a similar event from happening in the future, which is the ultimate goal of the team.

- **There must be a focus on standardized disciplinary standards within units.** This challenge is, by far, one of the most difficult to overcome. Ensure that fair standards, with a focus on the commitment to strive toward accomplishing organizational goals and objectives, have been developed and that all staff are aware of them from the first day of employment. Assure staff that there is a fair process that does hold them accountable for their actions. It should be understood that when an error is made, sometimes all an employee needs is counseling and/or coaching and to be reminded of a particular procedure or protocol. However, if behavior does not change and a similar event occurs, then the next step in the disciplinary process will be initiated and such action will be nonnegotiable. Managers also need to understand that when discipline is applied without consistency, it definitely lowers morale, leads to less respect for the supervisor, and can lead to grievances being filed. Remember that staff expect to be treated uniformly and that in similar situations, the same rules apply.

- **Leadership must walk the walk.** Staff will need constant reassurance that leadership's commitment is genuine and sustained. Patient safety and just culture training can be provided every day to the frontline staff, but if they don't see leaders change their own approach, frontline staff will not continue to put forth the effort to do the same.

                                       Creating a Just Culture

Putting In the Time

The most important thing to remember is that change is not instantaneous. This process takes months, if not years, before a full transformation takes place, and staff members will need to continually be reminded of this as the process becomes an integral part of the organization's culture. Because they are more conceptual in nature than, say, following a clinical pathway for pneumonia, quality, risk, and patient safety concepts and efforts have always been slow to take hold—but once they do stick and people understand why emphasis is placed on them, they are embraced.

To that end, leadership's commitment to patient safety as a strategic initiative is just as critical as staff buy-in. Just remember that because every organization is at a different stage in the quality improvement and patient safety process, patience is the key to slow and steady progress toward the ultimate goal of no patient harm occurring as a result of a medical error. Isn't that worth the struggles to get there?

As we continue our journey to drive a change in culture, in the next chapter we will be talking about benchmarking and how data can help drive that change.

Reference

1.   Reason, James. *Managing the Risks of Organizational Accidents.* Ashgate Publishing Limited, 1997.

 Creating a Just Culture

Evaluating Change

LEARNING OBJECTIVES

- Select the types of data that should be reviewed in order to support a safe and just culture

- Recall which steps should be taken for continuous evaluation of a safe culture

Would it surprise you to know that nursing has been interested in quality measurement since the 1850s? Florence Nightingale analyzed mortality data among British troops and actually reduced mortality significantly by organizing care and utilizing and teaching about simple hygiene. She is even credited with developing the very first healthcare performance measures. So as you may have surmised, nursing plays a most critical part in the delivery of quality healthcare, particularly in light of coordination with and integration of other disciplines. It is through this coordination that interception of most potential and actual events occurs and, for that, credit must be given where credit is due. On the other hand, nursing is also perceived, particularly when it comes to root cause analyses, to be the primary communication link between all healthcare providers, and when that communication link lapses for some reason, it causes leads to "failure to follow standard operating procedure" or "poor leadership" or "breakdowns in communication or teamwork," etc.

Much of the implementation of processes for transforming an organization into one that incorporates just culture concepts will fall to the nursing department, although eventually all departments will need to actively participate. That being said, although nursing will certainly play the dominant role, all units and departments will have an integral part in cultivating what are hopefully progressively positive outcomes as a result of the action items put into place. Once processes have been in place for a few months and baseline data have been disseminated to the staff, it is time to determine whether what has been implemented is making a positive impact on leadership's support of the initiative, whether the staff's behavior and the old perceptions about reporting adverse events are changing, and most of all, whether patient safety is becoming a primary focus throughout the organization. There are several ways in which this can be accomplished, but there is one common thread that must be included in the evaluation equation, and that is the use of data. Data tell a story, and if presented appropriately, can have a significant impact on the future of any project.

Data Are Necessary

Going back to the hot topic of falls, suppose staff members on a medical-surgical unit come to the risk manager and tell her that they are seeing an increase in the number of falls with minor injuries (bruises) on their unit because there is a shortage of patient care technicians (PCT) available during the evening shift to answer patient call bell requests for assistance to and from the bathroom. Unfortunately, no incident reports have been completed, even though staff members know they should have done so, because they don't want to be counseled for not watching their patients better. It now becomes difficult for the risk manager to bring this issue to leadership's attention because there are no concrete data available to support the need for additional staff members.

On the other hand, if staff members had alerted risk management of their concerns by reporting every time a patient fell because there was no PCT available and nursing staff members couldn't get to the room fast enough, the data could then be collected, analyzed, and displayed to reflect specific elements, such as time of day, shift, and any other documented contributing factors. This data could then be sliced and diced to best reflect the primary issues and the associated needs and then provided to leadership to support the need for additional staff members if, in fact, that's what the data regarding the main cause for the increase in the number of falls showed.

 Creating a Just Culture

Now, let's bring the rest of the organizational staff into the mix. They too will need to see what happens when data tell a story, so let's include a nonclinical example. An organization's emergency department (ED) seems to have a continuing problem every weekend with getting patients who have been deemed appropriate for inpatient admission up to their assigned units within an acceptable time frame. This, in turn, backs up the ED waiting room and increases patient complaints. Many patients end up getting very irate or leaving without either receiving or completing treatment.

Data are the objective information needed to demonstrate the need for certain actions to be taken in order for the desired change to take place. Data aggregation helps identify problems, offers consensus on best practices and evidence-based medicine, and affords the opportunity to share information with colleagues and peers. By using an automated or electronic reporting system, data collection, analysis, and reporting can be simplified. However, there does need to be a systematic approach to data collection, and data can be collected via a multitude of ways—through chart reviews, incident reports, lawsuit and claims reporting, financial and medical record coding, surveys, and many other data collection activities. The Institute of Medicine recommends that a combination of narrative and coded elements be collected when it comes to what information should be provided about near misses and adverse events and should, at a minimum, include the following:

- The discovery—who and how the event was discovered

- The event—type of near miss/event

- Where, when, and who was involved

- Severity and preventability of the event

- Likelihood of recurrence

- Ancillary information—patient and product information, as applicable[1]

When staff members are assured that the data being reported will not be used punitively but instead to develop better practices of care, reporting will increase and staff members will begin to include more information than just those data elements listed above. Narrative data are just as important as (if not more important than) objective data because they can provide additional information pertinent to the circumstances surrounding the event (e.g., whether the event occurred at the change of a shift, whether there were a lot of visitors, whether there were students present, etc.).

Measuring Progress: Patient Safety Culture Instruments

What do we need to evaluate, and how do we do it? First, we need to evaluate how well the organization has acclimated to a patient-safety-focused approach to healthcare based on the baseline survey done at the very beginning of this just culture journey. This can be done via several avenues, such as:

- Making random phone calls to staff members at home during off-hours to ask whether they feel the organization is supportive of a just culture environment. Staff members are likely to respond more honestly if they are not at work.

- Sending a brief survey via mail or e-mail and asking that the response be sent back by a specific deadline. Again, this allows for anonymity, and staff members will be more honest on paper and the rate of response return will be much higher.

- Convene a focus group.

For any of the above options, consider what questions should be included in this follow-up survey. Figure 6.1 provides some suggestions of questions to ask, divided into categories based on core indicators.

FIGURE
6.1

Measuring progress with patient safety culture instruments

Consider what questions should be included in your follow-up survey. Some suggestions would be the following, divided into categories based on the following core indicators:

Organizational Commitment	• Have the organization and senior leadership identified patient safety as a core value? • Do they support ensuring that there are adequate resources necessary for staff development and patient education on patient safety?
Managerial Involvement	• Is your manager or immediate supervisor supportive of patient safety initiatives? • Is he/she supportive if an error is made, and is it reported in a timely manner?
Employee Empowerment	• Do you feel you have been empowered to promote patient safety and prevent patient harm by taking responsibility for ensuring safe operations during your shift? • Do you feel you have a voice in patient safety decisions?
Accountability System	• Do you feel the organization has a fair evaluation and reward system to promote patient safety and discourage inappropriate or unacceptable behavior? • Is this system consistently applied to all hospital personnel?
Reporting System	• Do you feel the organization has a systematic and structured event reporting system? • Do you feel the organization has a fair incident/adverse event reporting system that is used comfortably by the staff?

Adapted from "Measuring A Just Culture In Healthcare Professionals: Initial Survey Results," presented by Terry L. von Thaden, Aviation Human Factors Division, University of Illinois at Urbana-Champaign, Savoy, IL, & Michelle Hoppes, The Risk Management & Patient Safety Institute, Lansing, MI, at the Safety Across High-Consequence Industries Conference, St. Louis, MO, September 20–22, 2005.

Resurvey Process

Once the survey tool has been developed, the organization needs to determine who will implement and own the resurvey process, as well as what will be done with the data once survey results start being reported back, then collected and analyzed. Remember that the entire staff needs to have feedback regarding progress made to date—if findings are not communicated back to the employees as well as to leadership, there is no way for progress to be maintained, nor will staff know whether their efforts have made a difference in regard to keeping patients safe. Of course, the best-case scenario is that the survey findings will show that the organization's culture of safety is changing for the better compared to the previous survey's findings, that findings are then shared with the entire hospital, and the culture of patient safety is moving toward a more patient-focused environment, not only for patients and their families, but for the staff as well.

Once staff begin to feel that such findings are an integral part of the equation for developing strategies to improve the organization's patient safety culture, the more likely they are to continue to take ownership of movement and the sooner that change will be more visible. Typically, results of the resurvey are mixed. Some units or departments will see improvement, others may not. For example, laboratory may see an improvement in its scores from the previous survey after implementing a change in staffing patterns that increased the number of employees on the evening shift, thereby reducing patient wait time in the ED because blood is drawn sooner and patients are diagnosed and treated sooner. They are also admitted sooner.

On the other hand, scores for leadership may remain the same if the staff still doesn't see them out there on the floors asking questions or encouraging feedback. But, be patient—positive change often takes time before being readily seen by others. What needs to be emphasized here is that if things aren't progressing as quickly as expected, leadership should seek the cause. In many instances, "work process re-design is a powerful component of the effort to improve patient safety."[2] Standardizing processes and protocols, reducing procedure redundancy, and utilizing human factors engineering techniques increases an organization's ability to get the patient the right care, at the right time, and with the performance of the right procedures. There have been many studies that show the more steps there are in a process, the more likely an error will occur.

The premise behind work redesign is to keep things simple. Make it easy to do the right thing and encourage teamwork. Tell staff to trust their own instincts when they think something is wrong and to take immediate action if they think it's necessary. Let staff know that you trust them when they tell you what needs to take place to make things better. Leadership must be committed to making the changes needed to improve patient safety, but it won't happen unless leadership truly is willing to make that leap.

Benchmarking

Benchmarking takes place at two levels. The first is the level of the organization itself, as it compares its progress from one measure of time to another. For example, if over the course of a three-month period an increase in the number of falls is noted (25% more than what has been seen in the past year), then obviously this notable trend should be investigated. Once a possible cause has been identified (say patients were given sleep medications at 10 p.m., and the highest incidence rate of falling was noted to be between 2 a.m. and 6 a.m., when patients woke up to go to the bathroom, as patients were unsteady on their feet due to the residual effects of the medications), action items to put into place should be considered. For this example, these might include pushing medication administration time to 8 p.m. and strongly encouraging patients to go to the bathroom before they get settled in for the night. Once these actions are put into place, the organization will begin to benchmark with itself every month/quarter to evaluate its own efforts to improve.

Benchmarking also occurs when the organization wants to compare itself to other hospitals. If so, then an already-established survey tool should be used, such as the Agency for Healthcare Research and Quality's (AHRQ) *Hospital Survey on Patient Safety Culture*. In response to hospital requests, the resulting data can be compared with that of other organizations by accessing the same, similar, and/or consistent tools, such as the AHRQ's *Hospital Survey on Patient Safety Culture 2010 User Comparative Database Report (www.ahrq.gov/qual/hospsurvey10)*. This report is published annually, and in 2010, more than 883 hospitals and more than 338,000 employees completed the survey. The report allows for comparisons between hospitals in regard to their patient safety culture. It provides data that will assist the organization with determining its strategic patient safety initiatives; it will also show the hospitals where they have improved, where they still need improvement and identify any patterns or trends that jump out and tell the organization of a definite need to investigate and evaluate further.

Some things of interest to note from the 2010 AHRQ resurvey findings are:

- Seventy-nine percent of the hospitals surveyed gave their hospitals fairly high marks for teamwork among staff members, indicating it was an area of strength

- Only 44% of the hospitals surveyed felt that their hospitals had a nonpunitive approach for staff reporting medical errors, indicating an area of weakness

- Fifty-two percent of the hospital staff members surveyed stated that they had not reported any events within the past year, and obviously this needs to be addressed

There is much more data in this report that an organization can access by going to *www.ahrq.gov*.

So, what do the above results mean? They mean that at the national level, in the 883 hospitals that reported their results to the AHRQ, progress has been made with respect to improving patient safety over the last five years, but we still have a long way to go before significant inroads are made to reduce the number and severity of the errors being reported.

Are more adverse event reports good or bad?

In regard to event report comparisons, there are things to consider when reviewing the data. First, there is the contradictory argument of whether an increase or decrease in the number of reports being generated during the monitoring period is a good thing. For example, if a 350-bed organization reports 300 incidents one month and then reports 350 the following month, leadership could conceivably say that the organization has a successful culture of patient safety, since the organization encourages event reporting. By the same token, if a 50-bed hospital reports 75 incidents one month and only reports 50 the next, it could also say that it has a successful culture of safety, in that the number of events has decreased because employees are empowered to be more patient-safety-focused, and therefore fewer errors occurred. Keep in mind that it's not necessarily the total number of incidents reported but, rather, it's the types of events being reported that need to be tracked.

Ownership of the event reporting process belongs to the department managers, not the risk manager or the patient safety officer. Each manager knows how his or her department operates and how staff members would best respond to change, certainly better than the risk manager or the patient safety

Creating a Just Culture

officer and, as such, must be responsible for following up on all reports to ensure that all issues are appropriately addressed and managed.

Additionally, each manager should be able to track and trend specific concerns identified. It is here that I think managers get the most bang for the buck—they can take a look at a cluster of events and dig deeper to see whether there are commonalities among them and, if so, can focus efforts on how to motivate change.

However, studies show that there is a definitive relationship between reporting rates and safety culture data. According to an article written in 2007 and published in 2009 in *Quality and Safety in Health Care* entitled "Trends In Healthcare Incident Reporting and Relationship to Safety and Quality Data in Acute Hospitals: Results from the National Reporting and Learning System,"[3] when staff members respond positively to questions relating to patient safety culture, indicating that they believe their organization is positively moving toward a just culture, they are more likely to report an incident, meaning incident reporting rates are higher.

Additionally, studies show that when staff were asked about their organization's overall scores relating to response and feedback about incidents reported, their responses were generally favorable and above the mean, suggesting that staff members get adequate responses and feedback from their managers but there is always room for improvement. In regard to accountability, from the staff's perspective, there was a huge discrepancy between the actions the clinical staff received versus the actions the physicians received whenever the error warranted attention.

What types of data should be reviewed?

It's critical to remember that incidents that resulted in harm, however minor, are not the only types of events that should be analyzed. Near misses, "close calls," and "good catches," as folks now like to say, should also be evaluated. Evaluating the causes of these types of common events *before* there is patient harm can provide valuable insight into what sequence of events led up to the near miss occurring and can provide a better understanding as to why particular actions resulted in an averted potential adverse outcome. In other words, you can answer the questions of what causal factors led to a patient almost getting hurt and what actions were taken to prevent the event from getting to the patient. Once these are determined, the focus can then be made toward developing and implementing methods and techniques to address them *proactively*. Taking preventive action will decrease the likelihood that any patient harm will occur in the first place.

When looking for valuable data to analyze, another avenue to pursue is claims data. Obviously, this is not a proactive approach, but this data absolutely should be reviewed for frequency and severity analysis, as well as the probable identification of a trend in specific risk exposures that should be brought to the attention of those most appropriate to take action as soon as possible. Failure to appropriately address these issues will, in all likelihood, lead to another patient getting harmed, and will also most assuredly affect future liability premiums.

Other data that risk and safety professionals may find useful in determining patient safety vulnerabilities can be found in patient complaint data; pharmacy radiology and laboratory data; all unexpected maternal or newborn deaths; unexpected returns to the operating room; returns to the ED within specified periods of time (usually within 24, 48, and 72 hours); readmissions within a specified periods of time; patients with long lengths of stay; and others. Administrator-on-call logs and administrative walk-around documentation can provide valuable patient safety information that risk managers and patient safety professionals can review to identify possible patterns and trends not otherwise picked up by the previously discussed data. For example, in my past experience as an administrator-on-call, I would be notified of any patient transferred from our hospital to another facility, which proved to be very helpful in ensuring that the patient received the best possible care before being transferred and that all Emergency Medical Treatment and Active Labor Act guidelines were followed. I could check that the transfer was appropriate and to a higher level of care that we could not provide, or at the patient's request, but not because of an attending physician's convenience, or because of a patient's past medical history, or because of the patient's ability to pay. I was able to document potential patterns or trends in the care provided by the medical staff, which would then be forwarded to the chief medical officer for further action.

Performance improvement data is also insightful in identifying potential patient safety issues. For example, if a patient was admitted through the ED with pneumonia, the Joint Commission's core measures data set for pneumonia requires that an antibiotic be administered within six hours of hospital arrival. Not complying with the requirements could lead to patients with unnecessarily extended lengths of stay; of course, the longer the stay, the more likely the patient is to develop an

 Creating a Just Culture

infection, a pressure ulcer, or some other hospital-acquired condition. Under the new Centers for Medicare & Medicaid Services (CMS) regulations, the development of certain iatrogenic conditions during a patient's admission must now be reported to certain regulatory agencies, and the hospital cannot bill them, if the event was determined to have been preventable. These data are collected, and those patient medical records identified as not meeting that criteria are reviewed and referred on to the appropriate medical staff reviewers, who will then discuss with the individual practitioner the need to follow the established protocols.

Use your data

Keep in mind that benchmarking on both levels—internally and externally—can and does provide organizations with information that helps them identify their strengths and weaknesses; however, in order for benchmarking to be an effective tool for change, it has to be acted on promptly and monitored continuously, or the exercise is futile and a waste of precious time. There are many organizations, groups, and regulatory agencies, as well as federal and state bodies that collect data, and from which data can be obtained for comparative analysis.

Such organizations include:

- Leapfrog

- The Joint Commission

- The Pennsylvania Patient Safety Reporting System

- Quantros MEDMARX®

- The Veterans Administration's Patient Safety Reporting System

- The University Health System Consortium

- CMS

- Individual state and local patient safety agencies and organizations

This willingness on the part of participating hospitals across the country to share these types of patient safety data lends credibility and validity to the efforts of individual hospitals as they strive to make their case for improved reporting and the development of improved patient care systems and processes.

Continuous Evaluation

Once you have evaluated change and benchmarked data to find areas for improvement, the job is not finished, nor does the organization stop its patient safety efforts. This is a never-ending process, and organizations must always continue their efforts to improve the quality of care being provided in order to promote patient safety and prevent patient harm. Organizations can ensure that patient safety efforts become second nature by doing such things as:

- Making patient safety an agenda item at every board meeting; at every quality, risk and patient safety-related committee meeting; and at quarterly medical staff meetings.

- Requiring the multidisciplinary participation of representatives from the medical staff, clinical and ancillary departments, as well as nutritional and environmental services on patient safety subcommittees, task forces, and work groups.

- Communicating analyses and relevant findings based on data review at every opportunity.

- Rewarding staff for participating in patient safety initiatives, letting them determine what those rewards should be.

- Tooting your own horns! When something is working, share it with as many folks as possible, and as often as possible. Praise staff for being innovative and willing to try new ideas, publish successes through newsletters, storyboards, posters, and flyers, or ask the information technology department to develop screen savers.

Once these data are collected, problems are identified, and solutions are developed and implemented, it is essential that this information be shared across the continuum of care and presented to all hospital personnel as well as to the medical staff, managers and department heads, senior

 Creating a Just Culture

leadership, and the governing body. By providing folks with feedback, whether positive or negative, staff is made aware of the bigger picture: the potential impact these types of events can have on the entire organization, what the impact was on the individuals involved, what actions were taken to prevent similar events from recurring, and what staff members' individual roles and responsibilities are in this process.

Through openly and frequently communicating with staff about patient safety issues on a regular basis, educating them about the organization's commitment to patient safety, constantly providing feedback regarding progress and the win-win philosophy of keeping patients safe from harm in a positive working environment, and holding everyone accountable for their actions through the application of consistent performance expectations for all those involved, the organization will send the message that patient safety is the first and foremost priority. The organization will create a reputation for welcoming the opportunity to change for the better.

References

1. Solomon, Ronni, and Simons, Sherri. Data for Safety Actionable Knowledge Tack Force. *Data for Safety: Turning Lessons Learned into Actionable Knowledge.* American Society for Healthcare Risk Management of the American Hospital Association, 2008.

2. *Leadership Guide to Patient Safety Resources and Tools for Establishing and Maintaining Patient Safety.* IHI, 2005.

3. Hutchinson, A., Young, T.A., Cooper, K.L., McIntosh, A., Karnoon, J.D., Scoble, S., and Thomson, R.G. "Trends in healthcare incident reporting and relationship to safety and quality data in acute hospitals: Results from National Reporting and Learning System." *Quality and Safety in Health Care* 18, no. 1 (2009): 5–10.

 Creating a Just Culture

Case Scenarios

- Recognize proven strategies from other hospitals for a successful just culture implementation

A Case for Public Reporting: The Maryland Patient Safety Center's "Safe from Falls" Initiative

The Maryland Patient Safety Coalition was initially established by law in 2001 following the release of the Institute of Medicine report *To Err Is Human* and, more specifically, after the death of 18-month-old Josie King due to a systemic sequence of medical errors at the Johns Hopkins Children's Center. Her mother, Sorrel King, and Peter Pronovost, MD, PhD, associate professor and medical director of the Johns Hopkins Center for Innovation in Quality Patient Care, a practicing anesthesiologist at Hopkins and a world-renowned patient safety proponent, were instrumental in getting the law passed and the center established to promote "the development of systems within Maryland healthcare facilities to prevent adverse events and enhance patient safety."[1]

Evolving into the Maryland Patient Safety Center (MPSC) in June 2004, with the Delmarva Foundation for Medical Care and the Maryland Hospital Association as its cosponsors, its purpose is multi-focused in approach—to provide education about patient safety to all who want to learn, to initiate working collaboratives designed to share and implement best practices in the delivery of safe patient care, to encourage the voluntary reporting of near-miss or "good catch" adverse events to the center for the purpose of collecting adverse event data, and to perform an analysis of the data to identify possible patterns and trends and then develop and implement effective, standardized strategies that will both promote patient safety and prevent patient harm throughout the state of Maryland.

In July 2006, the center introduced an online, Web-based adverse event reporting system that hospitals could utilize to voluntarily and confidentially report events without fear of reprisals; the data collected about these events could then be used at the hospital level to assist in individual facility patient safety initiatives, but could also be redacted, aggregated, and evaluated by the center from a more global perspective in an effort to possibly identify patterns and trends at the statewide level, with future patient safety activities planned based on what the data show. However, in order to promote voluntary reporting and in response to the hospitals' concerns regarding the discoverability of incident reports, the law afforded those incidents reported to the center protection from discovery, ensuring that all patient safety activities "shall be conducted by a medical review committee established under Health Occupations Article, §1–401, Annotated Code of Maryland." In other words, as long as the data submitted to the MPSC, which was considered by statute to be a "medical review committee," is used to "evaluate and seek to improve the quality of healthcare provided by providers of healthcare, [then] the proceedings, records, and files of a medical review committee are confidential [and] are not discoverable and are not admissible in evidence in any civil action."

After being assured that their data would be kept confidential and would be protected from discovery, six out of the 47 acute care hospitals in Maryland agreed to participate in the pilot, and staff members were educated about incident reporting. They were taught about why incident reporting was so important, that it is used to help identify potential patterns and trends that can be addressed through the development and implementation of patient safety strategies, and that the reports would not be used in any punitive fashion, although staff members would be made aware of any issues requiring individual attention.

Creating a Just Culture

Results after six months

In July 2006, incident report data began to be reported to and collected by the center. At the end of the year, approximately 800 incidents had been reported. These data were presented at the MPSC 2nd Annual Patient Safety Conference in Baltimore and revealed the following:

- Medication errors were the most frequent type of event being reported, with approximately 98% reporting no harm to the patient

- Falls were the second most frequent type of event being reported, with approximately 20% reporting that there was harm to the patient

A fall is defined as any unplanned descent from a higher level to a lower level, ground, or floor. Harm is defined as injuries that involve little or no care, formal intervention, or observation, such as abrasions, contusions, small skin tears, or minor lacerations that do not require suturing and that will heal within several days, to those injuries that are clearly much more serious and require medical intervention, consultation, or increased length of stay. These include fractures, head injuries with or without loss of consciousness, changes in mental or physical status, and death.

Because these data only reflected six months of activity, it was felt that the presentation could only report frequency and harm versus no harm and, as such, no definitive pattern or trend could be identified at that time. Data would continue to be collected for the next year and, at that time, it was anticipated that the data would be much more reflective of actual occurrences, and more definitive patterns could be discussed. At the MPSC 3rd Annual Patient Safety Conference in spring 2008, 2007 data presented included information contained in more than 5,000 reported events and, although there were only six hospitals using the system, there did seem to be enough data that could be considered representative of the types of events occurring in hospitals all across the state. The results indicated that:

- Medication errors were the most frequent type of event being reported, with approximately 98% reporting no harm to the patient

- Falls were the second most frequent type of event being reported, but now with approximately 24% reporting harm to the patient

Additionally, in the early spring of 2008, the MPSC received several phone calls from risk managers across the state asking whether other hospitals were reporting an increase in the number of fall-related malpractice claims. Furthermore, the Maryland Department of Health and Mental Hygiene's Office of Health Care Quality, to which hospitals are required to report what are known as "Level 1" events (those events determined to have been caused by a hospital's actions that resulted in serious injury, illness, or death, or conditions that lasted longer than seven days and/or were still present at the time of discharge), reported that falls were the most frequently reported Level 1 event.

Learning from others

Further research revealed that Minnesota had encountered a similar situation approximately two years earlier and had established a work group to develop a falls prevention program that was implemented as a statewide initiative, which was proving to be successful in at least preventing the severity of patient injuries sustained after a fall, if not the frequency of fall occurrence. Based on this information, a team representing Maryland hospitals and the MPSC went to Minnesota to visit the Minnesota Hospital Association and its patient safety staff to learn how they implemented their statewide program so that Maryland could undertake a similar initiative, as well as to visit hospitals that were reporting positive results. The team was very impressed with how each hospital visited was consistently following the standardized road map in regard to putting processes in place to prevent falls while still finding their own unique way of implementing and promoting individualized tools for staff members to use.

However, the one thing the Maryland team felt was missing from the Minnesota initiative was that long-term care and home care were not included. Realizing that falls are a universal patient safety concern in all healthcare settings, the team felt that the Maryland initiative should be expanded to include these settings too. With the information learned from the visit, the MPSC and the Delmarva Foundation for Medical Care collaborated with representatives from acute care, long-term care, and home care to establish a work group that would develop and implement a falls prevention program at the statewide level to encompass all levels of care. With permission, the road maps originally developed by Minnesota were adapted for use by Maryland facilities, and, along with materials and forms already being used by work group members, toolkits that included sample policies, procedures, and forms were introduced and made available to all participants. In return, facilities that agreed to participate in the initiative were first required to submit their baseline falls

Creating a Just Culture

data, which included information about both current outcomes and process measures, and were also required to evaluate their own individual falls prevention programs to determine whether processes identified in the road maps as being components of a successful program were part of their own.

It was hoped that by implementing the best practices included in the road maps that outcomes would improve, meaning the number and severity of patient falls would be reduced. Outcomes data were reported on a monthly basis, and process measures data were not to be reported for six months to allow organizations time to put into place those measures not previously included in their own programs but that were anticipated to improve outcomes once they were implemented. Outcomes data were reported on a monthly basis, allowing the facilities to see how they compared with the rest of the participants in the state (aggregate data sharing only). Initial participants included 28 hospitals, 14 long-term care facilities, and four home care agencies.

More falls, or more reporting?

What came next was, at first, surprising. When outcomes data were reported for the second month, the number of falls reported increased, although in most cases, no harm was noted. When outcomes data for the third month were reported, again, the number of falls reported had increased, although the rate of severity remained relatively unchanged. This caused the work group some concern, so during on-site visits to facilities to evaluate potential implementation problems, staff members were asked what obstacles they were encountering that hindered being able to prevent their fall frequency. It was then discovered that patient falls weren't really happening any more frequently than before the initiative was started—staff members just weren't afraid to report them anymore. Additionally, folks now had a clearer understanding of the definition of what constituted a fall and were now reporting more accurately. Staff members also realized that they were making a difference and being included as part of the equation to problem solving in regard to fall prevention. More notably, although frequency of reports had in fact increased, the number of patients reported as having sustained an injury was slowly but steadily decreasing. And this, of course, was the more important outcome.

At the six-month mark, when it was time to submit process measures data along with the outcomes, it was noted that compared with the baseline, compliance with recommended process measures had improved, and the number and severity of falls reported had decreased. As of this writing it's still a bit too early to confirm whether there is a direct correlation between the two, but clearly the implications are there. It is hoped that when the process measures data are resubmitted with the outcomes data, further continued and steady improvement will be noted, and the initiative may very well be considered a success.

Just Culture Reinvigoration: Medical City Dallas Hospital

Prevention of adverse events is a part of working in a hospital environment and, when an event does occur, how those events are dealt with can truly have an effect on patient safety. Because nurses make up one of the largest contingents of staff members, they are often involved in a near miss or medical error. Ensuring that your hospital's leadership team and upper management are committed to the just culture philosophy will help the nursing staff understand its role in error prevention.

Medical City Dallas Hospital (MCDH) addressed the need to involve managers by forming an executive council to review all potential near-miss and sentinel events, according to Laura Weber, RN, MBA, CPHQ, assistant vice president for quality and organizational development at MCDH. This process change is one of a few that MCDH rolled out in relation to sustaining a just culture over the past two and a half years.

"We reinvigorated our just culture process . . . and went back and talked about what a just culture is," says Weber. "We did training with our leadership group, with our board of directors, and with our PI/patient safety council, which is made up of joint medical staff members and hospital executive staff. By providing that education at this level, it gets spread to the rest of our hospital and medical staff."

The executive council that reviews all potential near misses and sentinel events goes over the definition of just culture with the meeting invitees: the staff member or members involved in the event and the manager of the unit where the event occurred, who has usually conducted an initial investigation. For more information on what types of definitions are reviewed with executive council, see the sidebar "MCDH Just Culture Definitions."

"This can be intimidating because the group is made up of our chief nurse executive, risk manager, vice president of quality, and myself," says Weber. "When we first started [this process], we knew what our intention was—to learn more about what happened and do the right kind of analysis—but [the staff involved] didn't know. So we had to do a lot of training on what the purpose of this council is."

 Creating a Just Culture

Using the principles of just culture, the executive council decides the next steps to be taken. This often involves performing a root cause analysis, dealing with the issue on an individual basis, or both.

Making 'believers' out of staff

At MCDH, there's an emphasis on balancing a nonpunitive culture with one that's completely nonblaming. Nevertheless, staff still need to be held accountable for their actions if high-risk behavior is discovered or policies are knowingly ignored.

"Process is usually your problem 98% of the time, but a just culture is going to make sure you look at the individual competency and behavior," says Weber.

Recognizing that human error will happen is essential to understanding why a just culture is imperative, she says. When reevaluating the hospital's just culture program, MCDH focused on three behaviors:

- Human error (e.g., mistakes)

- At-risk behavior (e.g., shortcuts, not following policies exactly in low-risk settings)

- Reckless behavior (e.g., conscious disregard for following policies and procedures in high-risk areas)

These definitions help the executive council frame its decisions on next steps, says Weber. If a safety event was the result of human error as opposed to reckless behavior, the course of action will reflect that.

Although meeting with the executive council can be a daunting experience after an error or near miss has occurred, Weber says it's at that point that staff members truly understand what it means to work in an environment with a just culture.

"Once they've been involved in that process, and certainly if they've been involved in a root cause analysis, that's when you make believers out of people," says Weber. "Because then they see that this was not punitive at all, it was really trying to figure out what went wrong and how we can prevent something from happening in the future."

Additionally, attending a meeting with the executive council shows staff members that the hospital cares about who it employs by going through the process of determining whether reckless behavior was exhibited—which is usually not the case, says Weber.

Seeing results from hard work

MCDH has found that having a broad focus on reducing errors and supporting a just culture has helped the facility maintain a low fall rate as well as a low medication error rate. Additionally, Weber says that since the hospital took a second look at its culture two and a half years ago, staff have rated the two patient safety questions on the annual employee engagement survey—concerning the reduction of medical errors and support for the reporting of patient safety issues—as two of the most favorably scored areas on the survey.

Advice for hospitals building a just culture

Continuous communication is a must if your hospital is serious about building and maintaining a culture of safety, says Weber. One of the areas in which MCDH has had to focus is making staff aware that they work in a nonpunitive environment.

"Even though we were doing it, we weren't saying we were doing it," says Weber.

Additionally, presenting real-life examples to the staff to demonstrate how easily adverse events can occur helps them understand the culture. It also shows that the organization wants those events to be reported so that a proper analysis can be done; however, this takes time and effort.

Involving staff members in the analysis of an event when something goes wrong has bolstered MCDH's efforts in sustaining a just culture. Through the executive council's guidance and process, the hospital has incorporated staff in this important process. But prior to the improvement project, Weber's team found that it wasn't involving frontline caregivers as much as it should have, she says. It took a recommitment from senior leadership to communicate the expectation that staff involved in the event should participate in the analysis of that event.

"That occurred on two levels. One, it was making the managers accountable for getting their staff to the team meetings and working with them on whatever they needed to do," says Weber. The second included working around night staff's schedules.

     Creating a Just Culture

MCDH Just Culture Definitions

The following definitions are reviewed in a meeting between MCDH's executive council and staff involved in a near miss or adverse event:

- **Close call:** An unplanned occurrence that does not cause injury or harm to people or property but, under different circumstances, could have.

- **Just culture:** Marx's four concepts of behavior create the link between the discipline process and patient safety:

    - **Human error:** Inadvertent action that caused or could have caused an undesirable outcome

    - **Negligent conduct:** System failure or failure to act as a reasonably prudent person (e.g., nurse, respiratory therapist) would have in the same or similar circumstance and that is directly related to harm

    - **Reckless conduct:** Conscious disregard for a substantial risk

    - **Intentional rule violation:** Intentional, knowing violation of a rule, procedure, or duty in the course of performing a task

- **Sentinel event:** An unexpected occurrence involving death or serious physical or psychological injury, or the risk thereof. Serious injury specifically includes loss of limb or function. The phrase "or the risk thereof" includes any process variation for which a recurrence would carry a significant chance of a serious adverse outcome. Major permanent loss of function means sensory, motor, physiologic, or intellectual impairment not present on admission requiring continued treatment or lifestyle change.

- **Serious preventable adverse event:** Any event (including Centers for Medicare & Medicaid Services [CMS] reportable events, CMS hospital-acquired conditions including those specified as serious preventable events, and National Quality Forum and Leapfrog serious reportable events) within the control of a provider that result in harm and require a new or modified physician order for management of the patient's medical care.

How Mistakes Happen: A Personal Medication Error Story

It was halfway through the evening shift in the ICU step-down when one of my two patients went into cardiac arrest. I remained at the bedside while the team began to arrive, staying completely focused on the events in front of me. As the situation began to stabilize, I stepped aside to answer the unit telephone. The physician on the phone requested that I take a telephone order for IV push heparin on my other patient. Without hesitation, I listened to the telephone order from the physician and then immediately returned to the emergency that was still in progress.

When the code situation was stabilized and the unit returned to a calmer environment, I knew I now had to follow through with the telephone order I took on my second patient. Because I was busy with the emergency and hadn't yet carried out the telephone order, I felt my priority was to first administer the IV medication as ordered. I proceeded to draw up the heparin dose, knowing that I could easily write the telephone order in the physicians' order book after the medication was administered.

I held up the syringe containing the heparin and, as per protocol, asked my coworker to double-check the dosage I had drawn up. I clearly remember looking at the syringe with the 9,000 units of heparin and saying to my colleague: "The usual bolus dose of heparin is 5,000 units to 7,500 units. Isn't 9,000 units a bit high?" My colleague responded, "Well, yes, but the physician must have his reasons...go ahead and give it."

So I pushed the 9,000 units of heparin and then went to the physicians' order book to write down the telephone order as I remembered it. I dated and timed the order, writing: "9,000 units of heparin IVP × 1 now."

As soon as I signed my name to the telephone order, I immediately felt a cold sweat and a panic set in. I instantly knew my mistake: The physician hadn't said "9,000 units," he said "900 units of heparin." But it was too late. I had already administered the incorrect dosage of heparin.

 Creating a Just Culture

Looking back, I clearly see everything I did wrong:

- I took an order over the telephone for a medication, but I listened only. I never wrote down and read back the order for confirmation.

- I took a phone order when in fact telephone orders should be reserved for emergencies only, or eliminated entirely with the advent of computerized physician order entry.

- I gave a medication without the benefit of having a pharmacist review the order for accuracy and allergies.

- Although I did ask a second registered nurse to confirm the dosage of the medication I had drawn up, neither one of us remembered to check for the very important corresponding lab value.

Everything I did was with the right intention, but nothing was correct because I bypassed every safety protocol that could have prevented my error. Luckily, the patient survived my mistakes because, in this case, an antidote could be administered.

This incident took place 20 years ago and it still feels like it was just yesterday. Have I learned from my error? Absolutely, and I have never repeated a similar type of error because the memory is too strong. But, thankfully, 20 years later, there are a lot more systems in place that can help a clinician administer medications without making errors.

— Gayla Jackson, RN, BSN

Reference

1. Maryland Patient Safety Center, *www.marylandpatientsafety.org.*

 Creating a Just Culture

Disclosure

- Identify cultural barriers to appropriate disclosure

- Identify who should disclose an error

Even in those organizations with the most supportive just culture and patient-focused delivery-of-care systems, healthcare providers are still only human beings, and adverse events will still happen. However, by reporting them to the appropriate individuals, determining the causes, developing action plans, and evaluating plan effectiveness, we hope to prevent similar events from happening in the future. Despite the best of intentions, when an event occurs that results in harm to the patient, it isn't just the patient and/or the family affected in the aftermath—the healthcare provider(s) involved can be just as distressed emotionally, or even devastated, particularly if the resulting harm has long-term or permanent effects on the patient or if, in the worst-case scenario, the patient dies.

There are several initial reactions a healthcare professional could have. One is to pretend it didn't happen or that it wasn't that serious, or that sometimes, despite the best intentions, bad outcomes happen, but it doesn't mean anyone did anything wrong; at the opposite end of the spectrum, the healthcare professional could blame others or blame him or herself and feel immense remorse or guilt. No matter what the initial reaction is, the first thing that absolutely needs to be managed as quickly as possible is communicating with the patient and the family. Specifically, what to tell them, how best to approach them, and who else should be included in the conversation must be thought about and decided upon before that first conversation takes place.

Per Joint Commission standards, under the patient rights section, "Patients and, when appropriate, their families are informed about the outcomes of care, treatment, and services that have been provided, including unanticipated outcomes." This means that when an adverse outcome occurs, and decisions about further care will significantly impact patients and their families, healthcare providers must let them know about the event and what, if any, additional care will need to be provided. Additionally, the doctrine of informed consent requires that patients be provided with information relating to the risks, benefits, and alternatives to proposed treatment, as well as the option of no treatment at all. In fact, informed consent is required by every state's law relevant to the issue, and it is to take place before any interventional procedure is performed, regardless of the original cause of injury, illness, or condition, iatrogenic or otherwise.

That being said, how an adverse event is communicated to the patient and family will more often than not dictate how the patient and family will react to the disclosure. Although from an ethical and moral, if not legal, perspective, disclosure of an unanticipated outcome should definitely be communicated by the provider to the appropriately involved individuals in as open and timely a manner as is reasonable; it also shouldn't be made without some careful consideration, not only with respect to the patient's/family's needs, but also to those of the healthcare provider. For many healthcare professionals, fear of the unknown can have a huge impact on whether to disclose or how much information should be communicated—fear that the family could react by being threatening physically or by being so emotionally distraught that consolation is just not possible, fear that colleagues will no longer trust them to provide safe care, or fear that any apology will be misconstrued as an acceptance of blame/responsibility and ultimately lead to a medical malpractice action.

Cultural Barriers

Other issues to consider are what the patient–provider relationship was before the event, as well as barriers to communication, such as language, physical disabilities, patient or family cultural and educational background, ability to comprehend what is being discussed, etc.

If the patient and the care provider have at least met and/or have an already-established relationship, then the extent of the relationship needs to be taken into consideration prior to disclosing, because it is usually easier for the healthcare professional to initiate a meaningful conversation about what happened if he or she has developed some sort of working relationship with the patient. For example, my parents had the same doctors since they were young adults, went to see them regularly, and followed their advice to the letter. For the most part, their generation considered their doctors to be the experts in regard to the care and treatment of their conditions and trusted that whatever the doctors said was for the best, even if the outcomes were contrary to what was originally expected. In fact, in some cases, they probably would have preferred not to know about anything that may have been unpleasant or difficult to cope with if it wasn't necessary or detrimental to their health or well-being.

Our generation, however, wants to be more knowledgeable about our conditions, particularly in light of all the information available to us via the television, the press, the Internet, etc.; we want to know about all potential outcomes, possible side effects from the proposed treatment, the benefits versus risks, and the possibility of alternative treatments, if any. In other words, we want to be included as co-decision-makers, if not the primary decision-maker, when it comes to what care is provided to us. The patient–provider relationship plays a huge role in determining whether disclosure about an event is the best avenue to take.

Additionally, Joint Commission standards require that the ability of the patient/family to understand what is being said is addressed. This requirement is another obstacle that must be addressed. If the patient's primary language is not the same as the provider's, or if there are physical disabilities that could hinder such understanding, then accommodations via an objective, third-party interpreter must be made to ensure the patient's/family's complete and total understanding of the issues relating to the care being provided, which includes the provision of sufficient information to enable the understanding as much about the occurrence of any untoward event as is possible and available.

Additionally, if the patient's/family's education is minimal or nonexistent, then medical information needs to be communicated in terms that are simple to understand, generally meaning that the provider must be able to communicate at a fifth-grade level.

Before disclosure can be made with honesty, integrity, and compassion, these factors, among others, must be taken into account and addressed with the appropriate individuals so that what is communicated is factual but thoughtful in approach.

The confidence to disclose is largely dependent on the culture of the organization. If a just culture is an integral part of the organization's beliefs and values, then the doctrine of disclosure has been included in every aspect of its patient safety culture, and every staff member, from the board to the medical staff to senior leadership to management and to the frontline staff, has been educated about, understands, and is in complete agreement with the components associated with the disclosure of adverse events.

Policy and Protocol

Obviously, there needs to be a formal disclosure policy, and it needs to include some fundamental components. From the beginning, basic terms need to be defined and a general consensus needs to be made regarding what specifically should be disclosed. ECRI's *Healthcare Risk Control Manual*, supplement "Disclosure of Unanticipated Outcomes," published in January 2008, and the American Society for Healthcare Risk Management's (ASHRM) *Monograph Disclosure: What Works Now and What Can Work Even Better*, Part 3, published in February 2004, provide definitions for the following terms: adverse event, disclosure, medical error, minor error, near miss, preventable adverse event, serious error, and unpreventable adverse event. Since these are generally accepted in the risk management and patient safety professions, they should be included in the organization's disclosure policy.

 Creating a Just Culture

Once definitions are established, the next decision needs to be which events should be disclosed, and should be in consensus regarding what should and will be disclosed. Some organizations feel strongly that all types of events defined should be disclosed, whereas others decide that only those errors that resulted in harm should be disclosed. Regardless of the decision as to what should be disclosed, all staff members, including board members, senior leadership, medical staff, management, supervisors, and frontline staff should be educated about the organization's disclosure policy and provided with clear direction regarding when it is appropriate to apply it and to ensure complete policy compliance.

To that end, the organization should provide some formal guidelines regarding how the disclosure conversation should be initiated, starting with acknowledging that an untoward event has occurred. The discussion should be initiated with sensitivity and empathy. It is probably at this point that the patient should hear an apology that the event occurred in the first place. The patient should then be told the truth, with a simple explanation that should include only the facts as they are known at the time, with no conjecture as to what could have or might have happened. No mention of blame should be made, and if the cause is not definitive, then it should not even be brought up. If the cause is known, then it should be explained to the patient along with the assurance that an in-depth root cause analysis will be conducted to determine contributing factors, develop action plans, and implement solutions to prevent a similar event from happening in the future.

I have always found it to be a huge benefit to all care providers involved if a "dress rehearsal" discussion takes place prior to meeting with the patient and family. This prepares the staff for what questions they should expect to answer and how best to answer them, both to ensure the patient's understanding as well as to ensure that what is said to the family will not put the hospital at risk for potential liability. Keep in mind that this is a very emotional situation for all parties involved, and that emotion needs to be allowed to be expressed, within some controls. There may be tears, anger, or even disbelief, and all of these feelings need to be acknowledged. If necessary, the patient should be either referred to or put in touch with the hospital's patient advocate, local clergy, social workers, and bereavement counselors, etc. At the end of the meeting, the outcome of the discussion should be validated and contact information provided so that additional questions can be asked and answered if necessary.

Following the meeting's end, a summary of the meeting needs to be documented, usually by the lead healthcare provider, and should include all people present and what was discussed. Where maintenance of the summary ultimately ends up, be it in the medical record or filed elsewhere, is an individual organization's decision based on the agreement of administration, risk management, legal counsel, the professional liability carrier, and whatever state statutes are in place that address the protection of peer review documents. Discussions with this same team need to take place with respect to whether waiving of current charges is appropriate or whether possible financial settlement should be considered.

Who Should Disclose?

Per Joint Commission standards, the "responsible licensed independent practitioner or his or her designee" should be the individual taking the lead when disclosing a medical error, and this should be encouraged as much as possible. Keep in mind that in an organization with a true just culture as part of its patient safety values and beliefs, the practitioner will have been educated and examples of how best to present the information to the patient/family will have been previously demonstrated to the entire medical staff, so that when/if the time comes, the practitioner will be as comfortable as possible under somewhat difficult circumstances.

In an organization in which a just culture is not yet fully embraced and the medical staff may not be as on board with the process, risk management should be ready and willing to offer immediate assistance to the provider whenever needed, including preparation beforehand and being present during the discussion. In the event that the provider refuses to participate in the discussion, the policy should include a back-up plan or "chain of command" process for disclosure to ensure a timely discussion with the family, regardless of who assumes the lead role.

Once that discussion takes place, additional actions will need to be taken with the provider who refused to participate, with the provider coming to understand that complete compliance is mandatory, not voluntary, and that noncompliance will result in disciplinary action, up to and including termination (of privileges).

It has always been my belief that happy patients don't sue. In my experience, in most cases in which a lawsuit has been filed, patients and families say they made the claim not because they felt that

© 2011 HCPro, Inc. Creating a Just Culture

someone was responsible for an injury, but because they felt that the healthcare provider didn't communicate with them about the circumstances surrounding the event. Additionally, patients usually don't distinguish between an "I'm sorry the event occurred to you" and "I'm sorry for causing the mistake to happen," so even if there is an adverse outcome, patients just want to be told the truth and want to hear an apology; whether there is actual liability or just an unfortunate outcome is irrelevant.

In many cases, if settlement was the best avenue of resolution, having been honest about the event right from the beginning can result in a more reasonable financial conclusion and a more satisfactory ending for all parties involved. The patient is reasonably compensated for his or her injury, and the physician has closure to a difficult situation that might otherwise take years to resolve. I am also a realist enough to know that some providers are much better at talking to patients and their families than others, particularly when it comes to discussing a very awkward and oftentimes complicated situation. Let's face it—some providers just do not have the greatest bedside manner, no matter how many attempts have been made to address it with them. To that end, ASHRM has published its four disclosure models to meet the needs of different situations as they arise, as well as to assist with determining which model best suits the circumstances at hand. A clear description of each can be found by going to *www.ashrm.org* and searching for "disclosure models."

The policy should also indicate where and by when disclosure should take place; usually within 24 hours is the recommended window of time by which providers should talk to the patient/family, in a quiet, confidential area large enough to comfortably accommodate all parties. That initial meeting will not, in most cases, provide an adequate or complete picture in regard to specifically why the event occurred, but it should include the fact that the event did occur and that there was an adverse outcome. Patients/family should know that a complete investigation into why this happened will be conducted and the patient/family will be updated regularly as to the status of the investigation; let them set the schedule for updates, if that is their preference.

Exceptions to Disclosure

On rare occasions, an event may occur that the provider feels just should not be disclosed to the patient or the family, because he or she feels that it would be detrimental to the patient's physical, emotional, and psychological well-being. Such decisions should be preliminarily discussed with representatives from administration, risk management, and legal counsel, as well as the chief medical officer or vice president of the medical staff and any other appropriate individuals, and then must be referred to the disclosure team as well as to peer review for further evaluation regarding whether the provider has acceptable reasons for feeling that it would be better not to disclose. Final determination by the peer review group needs to be documented, regardless of whether it agrees with the provider, and additionally, that documentation needs to be maintained, which is most commonly discussed in the committee minutes. Again, however, administration, risk management, legal counsel, and the professional liability carrier should probably be consulted to ensure the most appropriate place for documentation of this decision.

Resources Available to the Provider

Even though the organization has provided personal support to the provider and staff during the actual disclosure process, the fact that an adverse event with an unanticipated outcome occurred during the provision of care, services, or treatment can be a truly traumatic experience for all involved. Many healthcare professionals will need additional support that the organization alone may not be fully prepared to provide. Staff members should be offered the assistance of such professionals as social workers, clergy, psychiatrists, employee assistance program staff members, and bereavement counselors.

If more in-depth help is needed, additional referrals can be made through state professional associations, medical societies, and other healthcare provider alliances. Debriefing following the event will help the providers involved to decompress or at least share their initial thoughts and feelings with other members of the care team. If a staff member is having a particularly difficult time returning to work, allow him or her to use vacation or personal time to get away from the care setting for a few days, just so his or her perspective can become a bit more objective and he or she can return to work with a clear head ready to resume his or her duties. If the organization provides continuous support of a just culture and reassurance to the healthcare professionals involved that an honest environment of open communication is valued, providers will soon realize that by "talking the talk and walking the walk" in regard to a just culture, disclosure of an adverse event is the right thing to do for the patients who are being served by both the organization and its providers.

Nursing's Involvement in a Culture of Safety

By Terry L. Jones, RN, PhD

It has long been recognized that nurse managers have a significant role in moving the healthcare system toward a culture of safety. Recognition alone, however, does little to prepare nurse managers for this important task. The effectiveness of nurse managers in this endeavor requires that they understand what a culture of safety is, adopt its requisite values, and become equipped with the knowledge and skill to sustain cultural change. In other words, they need adequate knowledge, skills, and attitudes (KSA) to successfully achieve this objective. It is also important for nurse managers to view the role of cultural change agent as being inherent to and not separate from the role as manager. Such a conceptualization facilitates integration of activities aimed at cultural change with familiar management functions. Classical management functions applicable to the nurse manager include planning, organizing, staffing, directing, and controlling. The nursing work environment, which encompasses culture, evolves based on how these functions are carried out. Creating and sustaining a culture of safety can best be achieved by knowledgeable and skilled nurse managers through these functions.

The Current Nursing Workforce

The majority of practicing nurses today received their basic nursing education before 1990. This of course predates the landmark report *To Err Is Human*, which highlighted the myriad safety issues in our healthcare system. It also predates significant attention to a culture of safety in the nursing and healthcare literature. Therefore, few practicing nurses have been prepared by their basic formal education to lead the transformation to a culture of safety. Despite recommendations for the inclusion and emphasis of quality and safety content in nursing school curricula, wide-spread adoption has been slow. A recent review of top-ranked graduate programs in nursing revealed little evidence of dedicated patient safety content. Thus, even practicing nurses with a graduate education likely received no specific formal education in the area of patient safety culture. Given this gap in formal educational programs, nurses accepting management positions must assume responsibility for acquiring adequate preparation to perform this important aspect of their role.

Requisite Domains of Knowledge and Skill Sets

The first step in acquiring adequate preparation to create and sustain a culture of safety involves identification of the requisite knowledge and skill sets. Relevant knowledge and skill sets can be grouped into four main domains, which include the science of safety, culture, performance improvement, and management functions. Each domain, in turn, reflects multiple topics and skill sets as outlined in Table 1.

A careful review of the topics in each domain will help the nurse manager to identify potential gaps in his or her education and knowledge. Once identified, a plan to close those gaps can be formulated and implemented. At a minimum, the plan should include immersion in the related literature. A thorough review of the literature, through an Internet search engine, will expose the nurse manager to what the experts deem important. PubMed, one of the most robust databases in healthcare, can be accessed without charge. In addition, many organizations with an interest in safety provide access to seminal papers and bibliographies from their website (e.g., The Joint Commission, National Quality Forum, Institute for Healthcare Improvement, Centers for Medicare & Medicaid Services, Agency for Healthcare Research and Quality). Nurse managers should regularly search the literature and visit relevant websites to stay abreast of current knowledge. Nurse managers should also seek out opportunities to attend continuing education events relevant to the identified gaps.

 Creating a Just Culture

TABLE 1	Domains of knowledge and skill sets to facilitate transformation to a culture of safety

Domain	Topics/Skill Sets
The Science of Safety	• Natural Accident Theory
	• High Reliability Organization Theory
	• Human Factors Engineering
	• Work System Design
	• Complexity Science
Culture	• Organizational/Work Culture
	• Culture of Safety
	• Subcultures of Safety
	• Culture of Blame
	• Just Culture
	• Cultural Assessment
	• Cultural Change
Performance Improvement	• Frameworks for Quality Assessment
	• Performance Measurement
	• Performance Improvement Methods (PDSA)
	• Root Cause Analysis
	• Failure Modes and Effects Analysis
	• Error Reporting Systems
	• Data Analysis
	• Endorsed Safe/Best Practices
Management	• Planning
	• Organizing
	• Staffing
	• Directing
	• Controlling

The science of safety

A solid knowledge base in the science of safety affords the nurse manager an understanding of

leading theories about how and why errors occur, as well as principles of system design that facilitate

error reduction. Armed with this understanding, nurse managers are better equipped to design and manage systems in such a way as to significantly reduce errors and, in so doing, promote a safer environment for patients and families. The leading theories about error include natural accident theory and high reliability organization theory. Although these theories differ with respect to the inevitability of errors and mechanisms for reduction, the emphasis on system factors as the primary etiology of error is a key similarity. In both theories, the complexity of healthcare organizations and systems is recognized as a key factor contributing to error, and the inherent fallibility of humans is acknowledged. Both paradigms direct the nurse manager to look for inadequate system design or system failure rather than bad people when investigating errors. Likewise, these theories direct the nurse manager to design and/or redesign equipment and work processes based on current knowledge of human factors and work systems. Knowledge of human factors and related work design principles enable nurse managers to design the work of nursing to "fit" inherent human preferences and limitations, and, consequently, to reduce the probability of error.

Culture

If nurse managers are to transform culture, they must understand what culture is and how it evolves. Culture is generally described in terms of a homogenous set of beliefs, values, and assumptions that guide behavior within a social setting. Fundamental to understanding culture is the recognition that it is both observable and invisible. Although beliefs, assumptions, and values cannot be seen, the resulting behaviors and artifacts (constructed physical and social events) are quite observable. These aspects of culture generate the rules that govern behavior and become, in essence, a social contract that members accept. Cultural rules exist in both implicit and explicit form, and can be seemingly incongruent.

When applied to the workplace, culture is said to reflect assumptions about work ends and means—that is, what gets done and how it gets done. Organizational culture is "how we do things around here." Within the work culture, the basis for motivation and the strongest driver of behavior are assumptions about reward, i.e., people work in a way that is believed to result in some kind of reward. Human resource processes thus become the practical means by which a work culture is supported. Fundamental to the understanding of work culture is recognition of the existence of organizational subcultures. Subgroups (which may evolve based on membership in a clinical discipline, job category, departmental unit, or work shift) may develop differing expectations and assumptions resulting in different rules that guide behavior. Thus, interaction among these sub-cultures may yield conflict, unmet expectations, and uncoordinated workflows.

Our conceptualization of a culture of safety is built on a foundational knowledge of culture in general, and culture in the workplace. The safety culture of an organization is described as "the product of individual and group values, attitudes, perceptions, competencies, and patterns of behavior that determine the commitment to, and the style and proficiency of, an organization's health and safety management."[1] At the most fundamental level, safety culture reflects the extent to which safety is prioritized relative to other organizational imperatives such as efficiency, cost, and effectiveness. When safety is valued, certain visible behaviors and artifacts should be evident. Based on our understanding of the science of error and work culture, this generally includes proper-ties such as leadership commitment, positive and effective team relations, adoption of evidence-based practice, open communication patterns, organizational learning, a just approach to error management, and patient-centered care. In contrast, when safety is not valued as a top priority, or in the absence of a good understanding of the science of error, a very different culture evolves. An example of such a culture is that characterized as a "culture of blame." The differences in beliefs, assumptions, values, and artifacts between the culture of safety and the culture of blame have been clearly delineated in the literature. In contrast to a culture of safety, in a culture of blame cost containment is prioritized over safety, all errors are human errors, and patient safety reports are used for disciplinary action rather than learning.

Culture has also been characterized as "a learned product of group experience," which emphasizes that if culture is learned it can also be changed.[2] Although culture change is possible, it evolves slowly over time and does not come easily. Multiple barriers to creating and sustaining a culture of safety in today's healthcare systems have been identified. Akins and Cole describe these barriers as being systemic in nature, multidimensional (human, organizational, and technologic), and rooted in organizational policies.[3] They further contend that each of these dimensions must be addressed simultaneously in order to effectively improve patient safety. Common barriers include lack of leadership engagement, competing priorities and scarce resources, punitive culture and fear of litigation, resistance to change, and inadequate education about the science of safety.

Creating and sustaining a culture of safety involves removing barriers to cultural change, implementing strategies to facilitate cultural change, and assessing for evidence of cultural change. Although there are common cultural trends among healthcare organizations with respect to safety, organizations within the healthcare system proper and units within the organization reflect heterogeneous microcultures. Each of these microcultures has a unique combination of barriers to overcome and capacity to adopt new processes. Strategies for change should therefore be developed to fit the unique attributes of each microculture. A baseline safety culture assessment is thus an important first step in the change process. This assessment facilitates identification of barriers and serves as the reference point from which future change can be measured.

Although the science of measuring patient safety is considered to be in its infancy, reasonably valid and reliable approaches have been described in the literature. Specific assessment survey tools are listed in Table 2. Tools that measure multiple dimensions of culture are advocated, as they facilitate development of focused interventions and, when repeated over time, help identify how change in one dimension may affect other dimensions.

TABLE 2

Safety culture assessment survey tools

Assessment Tool	Source
Hospital Survey on Patient Safety Culture	AHRQ (www.ahrq.gov)
Safety Attitudes Questionnaire	University of Texas – Memorial Hermann, Center for Healthcare Quality and Safety (www.uth.tmc.edu)
Safety Climate Survey	University of Texas – Memorial Hermann, Center for Healthcare Quality and Safety (www.uth.tmc.edu)
Patient Safety Assessment Tool	U.S. Department of Veteran Affairs (www.patientsafety.gov/safetytopics.html)

 Creating a Just Culture

Regardless of the tool used, it is recommended that an entire organization, as opposed to selected departments or units, be measured annually, and that steps be taken to ensure that the sample is representative of the organization. Response rates below 60% have been characterized as "opinions rather than culture"[4] and should be interpreted with extreme caution. Examples of publications reporting findings from safety culture surveys are available in the literature. These examples serve as good resources for nurse managers struggling with how to interpret and present the findings of culture surveys.

Based on the findings from the baseline safety culture assessment, potential barriers to moving toward a culture of safety can be identified and strategies for change developed. Examples of strategies used by organizations to successfully bring about cultural change can be found in the literature. Although no two organizations have used the exact same set of strategies and interventions, a few common themes emerge. In each organization interventions were targeted to facilitate the commitment of leadership to safety and to increase visibility of leadership among staff. Specific examples of how this was done include leader-led safety rounds and placement of safety at the top of all meeting agendas. Education was another common element among these organizations. Educational interventions were multifaceted and ongoing. The foci of education included topics such as the prevalence and science of error, techniques for error investigation and performance improvement, and effective communication skills. Education was provided for leadership and all levels of staff, and team training was often incorporated. An emphasis on relationship building was another common theme. This emphasis started with relationships among executives and extended to clinical teams at the point of care. Education on desired team behaviors and processes to hold individuals accountable for disruptive team behavior are advocated.

Quality and performance improvement

Issues of quality and safety have reached epic proportions in today's healthcare system. Nurse managers are uniquely positioned to help drive changes needed for improvement. A working knowledge of improvement science is essential for nurse managers in order to capitalize on this unique position. Improvement science provides an organizing framework for the study of quality issues, tools to guide analysis of performance data, and strategies for implementing and evaluating process change.

The traditional elements of quality assessment in healthcare include structures, processes, and outcomes. Structure is defined as the setting and organization of healthcare resources. Process is defined as the activities that constitute care and includes both technical and interpersonal activities. Outcome is defined as the end result, good or bad, of care processes. Good quality outcomes are assumed to result from good structures and processes of care. Processes are judged to be good to the extent that they produce desired outcomes. This presumed link between processes and outcomes of care serves as the foundation of performance improvement activities. In the face of suboptimal quality and safety outcomes, this framework directs the nurse manager to search for faulty care processes as the likely etiology. Likewise, when processes are redesigned, this framework directs the nurse manager to evaluate the effectiveness of that change through analysis of outcomes.

Though conceptually simple, the actual evaluation of variation in processes and outcomes can be quite complicated in the context of today's complex care environment. One component of improvement science involves the application of statistics and analytic tools to guide evaluation of this type of variation. Examples of these tools include process control charts, Pareto charts, and comparison charts. Another component of improvement science involves the application of targeted strategies to aid in the identification of processes that most likely contributed to suboptimal outcomes. Examples of these strategies are root cause analysis and failure modes and effect analysis. Finally, there is another component of improvement science to guide the implementation and evaluation of changes in identified faulty processes. These components of improvement science are combined to form a very structured step-by-step approach to improving performance, known as the FOCUS-PDCA process. This acronym stands for find a problem to improve, organize a team, clarify the process, understand process variation, plan an intervention, do the intervention, check the effects of the intervention, and adopt the change into practice.

Management processes and functions

The role of managers in organizations today, including healthcare organizations, typically encompasses activities related to the functions of planning, organizing, staffing, directing, and controlling. Through these functions, work culture evolves and can be evaluated. These functions determine what gets done and how it gets done, and produce artifacts that reflect the underlying assumptions, values, and beliefs within the culture. They are both the ends and the means of work. Interventions to create and sustain a culture of safety are therefore subsumed within these functions. The nurse

 Creating a Just Culture

manager's values and assumptions about safety will guide the decisions he or she makes within each function. Staff, in turn, will infer their manager's attitudes and values about safety from the artifacts produced. Thus it is important that the nurse manager engage in reflective thinking to clarify his or her beliefs and values about patient safety before making a commitment to participate in any cultural transformation initiatives.

Management is a continuous process and the inherent functions more iterative than linear, each serving as a feedback loop to the others. These functions are not distinct processes, but rather are interrelated and at times overlapping. Nurse managers should review these functions and use them as a guide when seeking to lead transformation toward a culture of safety.

Planning for Safety

Careful planning by nurse managers is required to promote and sustain a culture of safety. The planning function is a process in which proactive decisions about the work to be done are made. The mission, vision, and purpose of the work are established and, ideally, drive all other work-related decisions. This includes decisions relative to the who, what, when, where, and how of work. It also includes decisions relative to the identification and procurement of resources to support work activities. Short- and long-term goals are established and the necessary steps to meet the goals identified and prioritized. Policies and procedures should be developed to outline what is supposed to happen. Workflows that sequence work activities should emerge, and interdependencies should evolve. Necessary supplies and equipment should be identified and budgeted, and human resource needs should be estimated.

Safe practices within the work of healthcare do not evolve naturally; rather, they must be planned. Nurse managers seeking to support a culture of safety should therefore approach the planning process with intentionality. Safety should be the guiding principle behind every decision in the planning process. Organizational mission and vision statements should be reviewed as unit work activities are planned to ensure congruence. Work policies and procedures should be developed based on current evidence and knowledge of the science of safety. At a minimum, procedures to support specific regulatory standards (e.g., The Joint Commission, nursing boards) and endorsed safe practices should be developed.

Procedures for endorsed safe practices alone, however, are not sufficient. Individual policies and procedures typically address a singular component of patient care and the work of nursing. In practice, however, nurses apply multiple policies and procedures repeatedly throughout a shift to meet the needs of assigned patients. Patterns typically emerge in how these procedures are sequenced and integrated into processes of care, also known as workflows. Due to the nature of healthcare today, work processes in nursing are influenced not solely by nursing procedures, but also by the procedures and workflows of many other disciplines and departments. The multidisciplinary work-flows that have evolved on nursing units have been characterized as complex, interdependent, tightly coupled, and error-prone. Transformation to a culture of safety requires conscious work design.

Process design and redesign are therefore key components of the planning function for nurse managers. This aspect of the planning function should not be done in isolation, however, but rather should be approached in a collaborative and participatory manner. All disciplines contributing to and affected by a work process should be included. Further, input from those managing and those implementing the work processes should be solicited. The evaluation and design of work processes should be based on the sciences of safety and performance improvement. Two branches within the science of safety, reliability science and human factors engineering, are particularly useful for this activity.

Useful techniques from improvement science include process mapping, control charts, and rapid cycle improvement. When work processes are designed without attention to human needs and limitations, error-prone situations will arise. In the face of limitations and/or unmet human needs, individuals will adapt processes and procedures in nonstandard and not quite ideal ways. When seeking to design processes that do adequately account for human limitation, the interaction of five work system components should be equally considered: individuals, tasks, tools and technologies, physical environment, and organizational conditions. Design principles that address human limita-tions relevant to these components include decreasing reliance on memory and vigilance, easy access to timely information, simplification, avoidance of ambiguity, user intuition, constraining and forcing functions, and standardization.

The nurse manager also must plan for safety when procuring equipment and supplies. This requires that the nurse manager consider volume, functionality, availability, distribution/placement, and

 Creating a Just Culture

inherent safety features (e.g., ease of operation, constraining and forcing functions) in the planning process. When equipment and supplies are not readily available, staff will make adaptations (e.g., substitutions, work-arounds, delays in treatment, inappropriate use of other equipment) that may threaten patient safety. Accurate estimates of volume, easy access to storage for all shifts, and strategic placement of frequently used and shared supplies on the nursing unit will ensure adequate availability. Managers should have a good understanding of the functionality of equipment needed to provide care. Equipment should be used for intended purposes only—those for which intentionally designed. When a piece of equipment lacks a needed functionality, staff will improvise, possibly in ways that threaten patient safety.

Finally, managers should assess for built-in safety features in equipment prior to purchase. When possible, constraining features that prevent users from inappropriate operation and forcing features that ensure adequate completion and appropriate sequencing of steps should be inherent in the design. Color coding of pieces intended to fit together is also advocated.

Organizing for Safety

The organizing function is closely related to, and at times overlapping with, the planning function. The organizing function provides the structure to support implementation of work activities developed in the planning process. It is through the organizing function that relationships are defined, tasks assigned, lines of communication established, coordination of resources outlined, and decision-making processes identified. The organizational structures that result from this function contribute significantly to the safety culture of an organization.

Implementation of planned work activities requires the coordinated efforts of multiple staff within and among departments. The nurse manager must provide a structure for how work activities will be coordinated within his or her unit, and negotiate structures for how work activities will be coordinated with other departments. Key decisions in this process that impact safety include assignment of roles and responsibilities for clinical and nonclinical tasks. The nurse manager should review organizational structures to ensure that tasks have been assigned in a way that does not threaten patient safety. Non-nursing work activities have been insinuated into nursing job descriptions and continue to be performed by conscientious nurses when left undone by other staff. Time spent on non-nursing activities by nurses translates into time away from nursing care, and can often lead to issues of poor care quality and job burnout. Nurse managers should review job descriptions and practice patterns to ensure that nurses are not spending their time doing the work of other disciplines. This may require advocacy for additional resources in other departments, clarification and enforcement of job descriptions, and careful negotiation of process changes.

Establishing the structure for cooperative and interdependent work processes requires negotiation of various time structures. When nurses care for multiple patients simultaneously, these time structures may overlap and be viewed as competing. For example, time structures may have been negotiated such that surgeons round and write daily orders at 0600 before going to the operating room (OR) for the first elective case, administration of preoperative antibiotics for the first OR case are due at 0600, and morning shift report begins at 0645. This results in a unit routine of significant time-sensitive work activity at the end of the shift for the night shift staff. When excessive, competing time structures may result in a sense of time pressure and delayed and/or missed care. The nurse manager should assess existing time structures and manage conflicts as indicated. Competing time structures can be effectively managed through renegotiation of existing time structures, changing task assignments, or increasing staff resources.

In this example, the surge in work activity demand could be anticipated by examination of unit routines. Surges in work demand also may occur as a result of unexpected events such as multiple admissions and discharges, sudden deterioration in a patient's condition, or staff illnesses. Surges in work activity demand, whether the result of poorly negotiated routines or unexpected events, pose a threat to patient safety and must be managed effectively. One strategy for managing these kinds of workload surges that seems to be increasing in prevalence is the incorporation of certain aspects of functional nursing care into total patient care delivery models. In the total patient care delivery model, nursing work is organized in such a way that the registered nurse provides all aspects of nursing care for assigned patients. In a functional care model, nursing work is broken down into separate components (e.g., medication administration, dressing changes, discharge teaching) and each component is assigned to a different nurse. In a pure functional nursing model, patients are not assigned a single nurse, but rather multiple nurses depending on their care needs and prescribed treatments. In a hybrid model, patients are assigned to a nurse who provides total care with the exception of a small number of interventions.

 Creating a Just Culture

For example, the admission process for all patients on a unit may be assigned to a single nurse or to the charge nurse, who has no other patient assignment. These functional assignments may remain continuous or be utilized only during known periods of high work demand (e.g., day shift). A similar approach would be to schedule an extra nurse to help out over the lunch hours (e.g., 11 to 2). The extra nurse could be assigned by function or to temporarily assume the assignment of specific nurses sequentially while they take a lunch break. For the unexpected surges in workload, a charge nurse without other assigned tasks could be utilized, or when associated with deterioration in a patient's condition, activation of a rapid response team might be a good strategy. The nurse manager should evaluate the need for these kinds of organizational structures and implement strategies that best fit the need.

Communication patterns also are key aspects of organizational structure that impact patient safety. In a culture of safety, errors are discussed openly and often to enhance organizational learning. Communication of information relative to patient safety must flow in multiple directions. Staff must be able to communicate concerns to each other as well as to management. Using the above example of surges in work activity demand, staff should have a mechanism to notify appropriate individuals of the problem and request assistance from someone with the authority to provide needed resources in a timely manner. Likewise, the nurse manager must be able to effectively communicate identified issues as well as changes in policy and procedures to correct identified problems.

Lines of communication should be clear and accessible to all staff on all shifts. Staff meetings are an effective means of communication only to the extent that they are well attended and/or the minutes are distributed in a timely manner. Further, there should be a mechanism in place to facilitate multidisciplinary communication. Structures that have been recommended include team huddles, multidisciplinary rounds, shared progress notes, and standardized formats (e.g., SBAR). The nurse manager should ensure that such tools are not only available, but are actually being utilized. Team huddles and multidisciplinary rounds cease to be effective mechanisms of communication when members are absent due to workload, scheduling conflicts, or lack of commitment.

Organizational structure is also realized through the work of committees. Committees may be assigned tasks, may serve as vehicles of communication, and may serve as decision-making bodies. Committee membership should fit the stated purpose. In other words, members should have the knowledge, skill, and authority to do what is asked of them. If charged with redesigning a work process, members should be knowledgeable about that process and skilled in process design. If charged with peer review, members should themselves be competent clinicians knowledgeable of nursing practice as well as institutional policies and procedures. If charged with establishing staffing guidelines for charge nurses, members should understand the role of the charge nurse, related regulatory issues, and available resources. If charged with analyzing safety data, members should be well versed in the science of safety. If charged with implementing strategies to improve a measured outcome, members should be skilled in the performance improvement process. Finally, if charged with making decisions, members should be given the appropriate authority to do so and subsequent decisions should not be routinely overturned by other individuals.

Committee resources also should fit the committee purpose. Committee resources include meeting space, supplies, staff release time, access to consultants, and access to information (internal and external). Clinicians may not be well versed in process design, workload analysis, data analysis, the science of safety, or performance improvement methodologies. This hinders their ability to be effective members on certain committees and ultimately detracts from the credibility of the committee's work product (e.g., recommendations and decisions). Yet clinicians do have needed expertise in clinical practice that other members lack, making their inclusion on committees a necessity. Busy clinicians also may have difficulty leaving the unit to participate in committee meetings or may not be willing to attend meetings or complete committee assignments on personal time. Resources for skill development and work release time are essential to ensure optimal participation by committee members.

Members also must have timely access to information necessary to do the work of the committee. Depending on the committee this may include administrative data (e.g., financial, supply utilization, human resource), clinical outcome data, or scientific literature. Finally, if the committee is charged with implementation of a communication and/or education plan, it should be given a budget to cover the necessary supplies and perhaps administrative/clerical support. The nurse manager should evaluate the structure and resource needs of committees and intervene as indicated. Examples of committees that have direct relevance to patient safety include peer review, performance improvement, patient safety, staffing and scheduling, and shared governance. The level of commitment to a culture of safety is reflected in the adequacy of resources for these types of committees.

 Creating a Just Culture

Staffing for Safety

In the area of human resources, there is significant overlap between the planning and staffing functions. For the purposes of discussion, planning for nursing resources will be subsumed under the staffing function. Activities inherent to staffing are generally categorized into recruitment, retention, and scheduling of staff. The process starts with the identification of the number and skill set of staff needed to carry out the planned work activities. Once identified, staff must be recruited, hired, oriented, socialized, scheduled, and continuously educated. Each aspect of the staffing function has implications for patient safety.

The number of nurses needed to provide safe patient care continues to be the subject of much debate and is often a source of contention between staff and management as well as between clinical and financial administrators. Staff often perceives that administration prioritizes efficiency over quality. and cost-reduction strategies have been implicated in the evolution of excessive nurse workloads. Excessive workload has, in turn, been implicated in declining patient care quality.

Although research supports a significant relationship between nurse staffing and patient safety, it has not reached the level of causality and is not sufficient to prescribe specific nurse–patient ratios. Nursing resource requirements are affected by multiple interrelated factors related to characteristics of nurses (e.g., education and experience), patients (e.g., acuity), and the work environment (e.g., work-flows, autonomy of practice, availability of support services and equipment, communication patterns). These factors are dynamic rather than static and are present in a unique combination on each nursing unit. Nurse staffing principles that address these factors have been adopted by the American Nurses Association (ANA), and it is incumbent upon nurse managers to conscientiously apply them when estimating staffing requirements and implementing staffing plans. Up-to-date information on the principles of safe staffing, related issues, and related references is available from the ANA (*http://safestaffingsaveslives.org*).

Application of the ANA's Nurse Staffing Principles requires that the nurse manager consider all related factors when estimating staffing needs during the planning function and, once estimated, periodically assess for changes that might impact staffing effectiveness. The lack of adequate data on these factors has been a significant barrier to the application of these principles by nurse managers.

The absence of credible data to justify requested nursing resources places the nurse manager at a disadvantage during the budgeting process. Historically, quality and safety data sensitive to nursing care has not been readily available. Missed care and adverse events are not always documented and are underreported. Thus retrieval of this information is challenging and often costly. Although nurses may report that workloads are excessive, this information is often labeled "soft" data and has not been valued as credible evidence. Empirical evidence now suggests that nurse perceptions of missed care may actually be a better indicator of patient outcome than more objective measures of workload. Nurse managers should continue to collaborate with staff in other departments, such as finance and health IT to improve the quality of objective data available to support staffing decisions. They should also advocate for the use of subjective experiential data from the staff to support nursing resource requirements.

Decisions about how nursing resources are distributed across work shifts can be viewed as aspects of both the staffing and organizing functions. The nursing resource needs for a given shift are contingent upon how work activities have been organized (e.g., job descriptions and care delivery model) and how time structures have been negotiated. The impact of these decisions on work demand and patient safety has already been discussed as part of the organizing function.

The next step in the staffing process for nurse managers involves generation of a schedule. Schedules are typically generated based on unit trends in patient volume and acuity, characteristics and availability of unit staff, and established unit routines. Changes in any of these factors, individually or in combination, after the schedule is posted can result in inadequate staffing. For example, when there is turnover or staff illnesses, scheduled staff may be replaced with nurses floating from other units or less experienced nurses seeking extra shifts. In this instance the overall experience and competence level of the staff for a shift may change in a way that significantly affects productivity and safety. Nurse managers should ensure that there is a mechanism to assess these situations and a process for resolution when they occur. In-house centralized staffing pools have been advocated as an alternative to the use of temporary staff from external agencies to cover vacancies. Likewise, long-term contracts with individual nurses from external agencies are preferred over per diem contracts.

Nurse managers also must address the issue of staff fatigue during the scheduling process. Fatigue has been shown to negatively affect job performance and patient safety. Factors known to increase

Creating a Just Culture

fatigue include shift duration and frequency. This research has called into question the wisdom of incorporating overtime and 12-hour shifts in nurse staffing plans. It is now recommended that nurses not be scheduled to work in excess of 12 hours consecutively or more than 60 hours in a given week. Alternatives for filling staff vacancies must be in place to support compliance with these recommendations. Absent these alternatives, nurse managers are faced with the dilemma of weighing the risks of not filling a vacancy and filling a vacancy with a fatigued nurse. Certainly both pose some risk to patient safety, and there is little evidence to guide decision making in this context. Prevention is the best course of action, and nurse managers should be proactive in identifying viable alternatives.

Recruitment and hiring staff with the right skill set also is part of the staffing function. The right skill set for patient safety extends beyond the clinical skills required for a specific patient population. The nature of healthcare and the work environment today require that nurses also have skills in the areas of communication, conflict management, and teamwork. Nurse managers must be very intentional in the interview process to assess for proficiency in these areas. Behavior-based interviewing techniques are considered particularly useful to this end.

Patient safety is enhanced when staff are adequately oriented to their roles and their environments. Staff nurses have responsibilities related to their roles as providers of care and as employees of the organization, all of which must be covered in orientation. Although aspects of the orientation process may be delegated to others (e.g., nurse educator, preceptor, organizational development staff), the nurse manager is ultimately responsible for ensuring that staff receive an adequate orientation and are competent to practice within the scope of their job description and license. New staff should be made aware of expectations inherent in a culture of safety. Specifically, they should receive instruction on how to report errors and safety concerns and be encouraged to report as indicated. New staff should understand how to access information on policies and procedures and should know how to safely operate the equipment used on their assigned unit. They should understand the chain of command for resolving conflict encountered on their assigned unit, including instances of perceived unsafe assignments or physician orders.

Traditional clinical competencies (e.g., assessment, diagnostic reasoning, symptom recognition, psychomotor skills, selection and prioritization of appropriate interventions) are not sufficient for safe practice or for meeting all employee role expectations in healthcare organizations. Nursing staff also must be skilled in the areas of communication, conflict management, teamwork, performance improvement techniques, process design, evidence-based practice, and the science of safety. As discussed, these skills have only recently been emphasized in basic nursing programs, and continued development of these skills beyond graduation and initial employee orientation is essential. Team training has been advocated as an effective mechanism to enhance performance in many of these areas.

In a culture of safety, staff is committed to learning. Nurse managers should therefore work with staff to facilitate continued growth and development. This may require release time to attend formal programs (internally and/or externally) and perhaps financial support for registration, consultant, and/or speaker fees. Nurse managers must proactively plan for continuing education of staff and advocate for resources as necessary in the budget process. Estimates of resources for backfill of vacancies related to continuing education requirements are essential. With respect to team training, nurse managers must collaborate with colleagues in other disciplines and departments to create and coordinate opportunities for team learning. A credible commitment to learning cannot exist without dedicated resources.

Directing for Safety

The directing function is the part of management where plans and structures are actually put into action and for that reason also is sometimes referred to as the activating function. Directing is less about what work gets done and more about how work gets done. In this sense, directing reflects how a manager approaches and responds to the work environment and can significantly impact the invisible aspects of culture and the climate on a nursing unit. It is through the directing function that nurse managers motivate, communicate, collaborate, resolve conflict, build effective teams, and apply rewards and punishments for behavior. The nurse manager's personal philosophy, beliefs, and values about safety and error become particularly transparent through his or her approach to the directing function. When safety is truly a priority and error is believed to result primarily from faulty systems, a pattern of directing behaviors will likely be evident.

In a culture of safety, managers demonstrate a style of communication that is open and honest. They are approachable and supportive rather than punitive when informed of errors. They seek out

 Creating a Just Culture

information relative to performance on safety and quality indicators. Procedures and expectations are established with staff input and enforced consistently. Conflict is effectively managed rather than avoided, and crucial conversations about sensitive issues are initiated. Errors are consistently disclosed and evaluated for learning. Individual preferences are set aside, and change is implemented for the sake of safety. Rewards and punishments are applied consistently and are appropriate to the context. Collaborative problem solving and process design is initiated to improve reliability. Effective teams are built and empowered to make decisions and take action to improve quality and safety. Consistent demonstration of these directing behaviors creates an environment of trust where staff has a safe place to fall when mistakes are made.

As discussed, the system for reward and punishment is integral to a culture as it reflects what is truly valued. When a certain behavior is valued, it is rewarded when present and punished, or at least not rewarded when absent. Through the application of reward and punishment, normative behavior is defined and controlled. Inherent in this process is performance measurement, be it implicit or explicit. Managers and leaders in an organization play a crucial role in this process through the controlling function. Through the controlling function, performance is measured against some established criteria (goals, benchmark targets, standards, indicators) and corrective action implemented as indicated for improvement. In a culture of safety, learning for improvement is an inherent value. Mistakes are viewed as opportunities for improvement, and there is a strong drive to do and be better. Evaluation of performance relative to safety is not only necessary, but highly valued. A working knowledge of improvement science is therefore particularly useful for the effective application of the controlling function for nurse managers.

All levels of performance within an organization (e.g., individual staff, groups, unit, and nurse manager) should be evaluated for effectiveness. In a culture of safety there is emphasis on looking for system causes of error, but individual accountability is not overlooked. A "no blame" culture is not synonymous with a "just" culture. Blameworthy and blameless acts coexist, even in a culture of safety. Nurse managers must be skilled in differentiating between the two and must apply procedures for disciplinary action when indicated. Failure to address blameworthy acts will result in the willful disregard of rules by some providers and may negatively affect the overall morale of the unit. Additionally, state licensing boards require that certain categories of error and behavior be reported for further investigation. Nurse managers should be knowledgeable of and compliant with these requirements as well as internal policies and procedures for progressive disciplinary action.

As discussed, high-performing teams are essential to patient safety. Conscientious planning, organizing, hiring, and training for effective teams does not guarantee high performance. The conscious and intentional evaluation of team performance and provision of feedback to team members are essential to support growth and development of these skills and establish normative behavior consistent with a culture of safety. What gets measured gets fixed. Nurse managers should therefore be knowledgeable and skilled in the evaluation of team behavior. Tools to assist in the measurement and evaluation of team performance are available in the literature. Team outcomes as well as team processes should be measured and shared with team members. When a root cause analysis points to ineffective teamwork as the etiology of error, the whole team should receive feedback and participate in the development of a corrective action plan.

Nurse managers should ensure the availability of unit-level performance data relative to patient safety. Managers must be familiar with the error reporting system in their organization and be able to extract reports that facilitate a meaningful analysis of performance. When data reports are provided by other parties, the nurse manager should be diligent in his or her review of the data to ensure accurate interpretation. Knowledge of improvement science will help the nurse manager know what questions to ask about data reports and facilitate interpretation of statistics and graphs. Positive and negative trends in data should be identified and used for improvement. In the face of positive trends, the nurse manager should recognize and reward staff for high performance. The nurse manager should also share negative trends with staff and seek input regarding possible contributing factors. Strategies such as root cause analysis (RCA); failure modes and effect analysis (FMEA); and tools such as the taxonomy of error, root cause analysis, and practice responsibility (TERCAP) should be utilized to identify problems. Once likely problems are identified, the FOCUS-PDCA process should be applied to facilitate corrective action.

Finally, the nurse manager should engage in some form of self-evaluation. The value of a cultural assessment with respect to safety has already been discussed and examples of assessment tools provided (Table 2). The nurse manager should use the results of the cultural assessment to determine the extent to which a culture of safety has been achieved on his or her unit. Opportunities for improvement should be identified and strategies for corrective action integrated into the appropriate management function. High performance should also be recognized and celebrated. Nurse managers should share successes with peers and colleagues to facilitate organizational learning and help spread the transformation to other units.

Bibliography

Aiken, L. H., Clarke, S. P., Sloane, D. M., Sochalski, J. & Silber, J. H. (2002). Hospital nurse staffing and patient mortality, nurse burnout, and job dissatisfaction. *Journal of the American Medical Association, 288*:1987–1993.

Altunas, S. & Baykal, U. (2010). Relationships between nurses' organizational trust levels and their organizational citizenship behaviors. *Journal of Nursing Scholarship, 42*(2):186–194.

Ashley, L., Armitage, G., Neary, M. & Hollingsworth, G. (2010). A practical guide to failure mode and effects analysis in health care: making the most of the team and its meetings. *The Joint Commission Journal on Quality and Patient Safety, 36*(8):351–358.

Baker, D. P., Day, R. & Salas, E. (2006). Teamwork as an essential component of high-reliability organizations. *Health Services Research, 41*(4):1576–1598.

Battles, J. B., Dixon, N. M., Borotkanics, R. J., Rabin-Fastmen, B. & Kaplan, H. S. (2006). Sensemaking of patient safety risks and hazards. *Health Services Research, 41*(4):1555–1574.

Bargagliotti, L. A. & Lancaster, J. (2007). Quality and safety education in nursing: more than new wine in old skins. *Nursing Outlook, 55*(3):156–158.

Beckman, S. L. & Katz, M. L. (2000). The business of health care concerns us all. *California Management Review, 43*(1):9–12.

Benner, P. E., Malloch, K. & Sheets, V. (2010). *Nursing Pathways for Patient Safety.* St Louis: Mosby. Berwick, D. M. (2008). The science of improvement. *Journal of the American Medical Association, 299*(10):1182–1184.

Blumenthal, D. & Kilo, C. M. (1998). A report card on continuous quality improvement. *Milbank Quarterly, 76*(4):625–648.

Boston-Fleischhauer, C. (2008). Enhancing healthcare process design with human factors engineering and reliability science, Part 1: setting the context. *Journal of Nursing Administration, 38*(1):27–32.

Boston-Fleischhauer, C. (2008). Enhancing healthcare process design with human factors engineering and reliability science, Part 2: applying the knowledge to clinical documentation systems. *Journal of Nursing Administration, 38*(2):84–89.

Brunsson, K. H. (2008). Some effects of Fayolism. *International Studies Management & Organization, 38*(1):30–47.

Carayon, P., Alvarado, C. J. & Hundt, A. S. (2007). Work design and patient safety. *Theoretical Issues in Ergonomics Science, 8*(5):395–428.

Cesario, S. K. & Stichler, J. (2009). Designing health care environments: part II. Preparing nurses to be design team members. *Journal of Continuing Education in Nursing, 40*(7):324–328.

Cohen, M. M., Eustis, M. A. & Gribbins, R. E. (2003). Changing the culture of patient safety: Leadership's role in health care quality improvement. *Joint Commission Journal on Quality and Safety, 29*(7):329–335.

Committee on Quality of Health Care in America, *Crossing the Quality Chasm: A New Health System for the 21st Century.* Institute of Medicine (2001). Washington, DC: National Academy Press.

Cornell, P., Herrin-Griffith, D., Keim, C., Petschonek, S., Sanders, A. M., D'Mello, S., Golden, T. W. & Shepherd, G. (2010). Transforming nursing workflow, part 1. The chaotic nature of nurse activities. *Journal of Nursing Administration, 40*(9):366–373.

Crainer, S. (2003). One hundred years of management. *Business Strategy Review, 14*(2):41–49.

Cronenwett, L., Sherwood, G., Barnsteiner, J., Disch, J., Johnson, J., Mitchell, P., Sullivan, D. T. & Warren, J. (2007). Quality and safety education for nurses. *Nursing Outlook, 55*(3):122–131.

     Creating a Just Culture

Crowley, C. F. & Nalder, E. (2009). Within health care hides massive, avoidable death toll. *Houston Chronicle*. Retrieved from *www.chron.com*.

Cunningham, J. B. (1979). The management systems: Its functions and processes. *Management Science, 25*(7):657–670.

Day, L. & Smith, E. L. (2007). Integrating quality and safety content into clinical teaching in the acute care setting. *Nursing Outlook, 55*(3):138–143.

Dianis, N. L. & Cummings, C. (1998). An interdisciplinary approach to process improvement. *Journal of Nursing Care Quality, 12*(4):49–59.

Dickey, N. W., Corrigan, J. M. & Denham, C. R. (2010). Ten-year retrospective review. *Journal of Patient Safety, 6*(1):1–4.

Dixon, N. M. & Shofer, M. (2006). Patterns, culture, and reliability. *Health Services Research, 41*(4):1618–1632.

Donabedian, A. (2003). *An Introduction to Quality Assurance in Health Care*. Oxford: Oxford University Press.

Dziuba-Ellis, J. (2006). Float pools and resource teams. A review of the literature. *Journal of Nursing Care Quality, 21*(4):352–359.

Fayol, H. (1949). *General and Industrial Management*. London: Pitman.

Firth-Cozens, J. (2001). Cultures for improving patient safety through learning: the role of teamwork. *Quality in Health Care, 10*(Suppl II):ii26-ii31.

Fox, R. T., Fox, D. H. & Wells, P. J. (1999). Performance of front line management functions on productivity of hospital unit personnel. *Journal of Nursing Administration, 29*(9):12–8.

Frankel, A. S., Leonard, M. W. & Denham, C. R. (2006). Fair and just culture, team behavior, and leadership engagement: the tools to achieve high reliability. *Health Services Research, 41*(4):1690–1709.

Gaba, D. M. (2000). Structural and organizational issues in patient safety: a comparison of health care to other high-hazard industries. *California Management Review, 43*(1):83–102.

Galford, R. & Drapeau, A. S. (2003). The enemies of trust. *Harvard Business Review, 81*(2):88–95.

Gantz, N., Sorenson, L. & Howard, R. L. (2003). A collaborative perspective on nursing leadership in quality improvement. *Nursing Administration Quarterly, 27*(4):324–329.

Geiger-Brown, J. & Trinkoff, A. M. (2010). Is it time to pull the plug on 12-hour shifts? Part 1. The evidence. *Journal of Nursing Administration, 40*(3):100–102.

Geiger-Brown, J. & Trinkoff, A. M. (2010). Is it time to pull the plug on 12-hour shifts? Part 3. Harm reduction strategies if keeping 12-hour shifts. *Journal of Nursing Administration, 40*(9):357–359.

Gelinas, L. S. & Loh, D. Y. (2004). The effect of workforce issues on patient safety. *Nursing Economics, 22*(5):266–279.

Ginsburg, L. R., Chuang, Y., Berta, W. B., Norton, P. G., Tregunno, D. & Richardson, J. (2010). The relationship between organizational leadership for safety and learning from patient safety events. *Health Services Research, 43*(3):607–632.

Grol, R., Baker, R. & Moss, F. (2002). Quality improvement research: Understanding the science of change in health care; essential for all who want to improve health care. *Quality and Safety in Health Care, 11*(2):110–112.

Grosbee, J. W. (2005). *Using Human Factors Engineering to Improve Patient Safety*. Oakbrook Terrace, IL: Joint Commission Resources.

Grout, J. R. (2006). Mistake proofing: changing designs to reduce error. *Quality and Safety in Health Care, 15*(Suppl I):i44-i49.

Haig, K. M., Sutton, S. & Whittington, J. (2006). SBAR: A shared mental model for improving communication between clinicians. *The Joint Commission Journal on Quality and Patient Safety, 32*(3):167–175.

Hall, L. W., Moore, S. M. & Barnsteiner, J.H. (2008). Quality and nursing: Moving from a concept to a core competency. *Urologic Nursing, 28*(6):417–425.

Hamm, J. (2006). The five messages leaders must manage. *Harvard Business Review, 84*(5):115–123.

Hansen, M. M., Durbin, J., Sinkowitz, R., Vaughn, A., Langowski, M. & Gleason, S. (2003). Do no harm: Provider perceptions of patient safety. *Journal of Nursing Administration, 33*(10):507–511.

Hartmann, C. W., Meterko, M., Rosen, A. K., Zhao, S., Shokeen, P., Singer, S. & Gaba, D. M. (2009). Relationship of hospital organizational culture to patient safety climate in the Veterans Health Administration. *Medical Care Review, 66*(3):320–338.

Hatler, C., Milton, D. & Clark, C. (1999). Methodological issues in performance improvement in integrated systems. *Journal of Nursing Care Quality, 13*(3):47–58.

Henderson, D., Carson-Stevens, A., Bohnen, J., Gutnik, L., Hafiz, S. & Mills, S. (2010). Check a box. Save a life: How student leadership is shaking up health care and driving a revolution in patient safety. *Journal of Patient Safety, 6*(1):43–47.

Hendrich, A., Chow, M. P. & Goshert, W. S. (2009). A proclamation for change. Transforming the hospital patient care environment. *Journal of Nursing Administration, 39*(6):266–275.

Howard, J. N. (2010). The missing link: Dedicated patient safety education within top-ranked nursing school curricula. *Journal of Patient safety, 6*(3):165–171.

Jones, T. L. (2010). A holistic framework for nursing time: Implications for theory, practice, and research. *Nursing Forum, 45*(3):185–196.

Hyun, S., Bakken, S., Douglas, K. & Stone, P. W. (2008). Evidence-based staffing: Potential roles for informatics. *Nursing Economics, 26*(3):151–173.

(The) Joint Commission. (2010). 2010 National Patient Safety Goals. Retrieved from *www.jointcommission.org/patientsafety/nationalpatientsafetygoals/* on October 27, 2010.

Kaissi, A. (2006). An organizational approach to understanding patient safety and medical errors. *Health Services Research, 25*(4):292–305.

Kalisch, B. J. (2008). The effects of consistent nursing shifts on teamwork and continuity of care. *Journal of Nursing Administration, 38*(3):132–137.

Kalisch, B. J. & Aebersold, M. (2010). Interruptions and multitasking in nursing care. *The Joint Commission Journal on Quality and Patient Safety, 36*(3):126–132.

Kessler, R. (2006). *Competency-Based Interviews.* Franklin Lakes, NJ: Career Press.

Kilgore, R. V. & Langford, R. W. (2009). Reducing the failure risk of interdisciplinary healthcare teams. *Critical Care Nursing Quarterly, 32*(2):81–88.

Kohn, L. T., Corrigan, J. M. & Donaldson, M. S. (2000). To Err Is Human: Building a Safer Health System. Committee on Quality of Health Care in America. Washington, DC: National Academy Press.

Lageson, C. (2004). Quality focus of the first line manager and relationship to unit outcomes. *Journal of Nursing Care Quarterly, 19*(4):336–342.

Landrigan, C. P., Czeisler, C. A., Barger, L. K., Ayas, N. T., Rothschild, J. M., & Lockley, S. W. (2007). Effective implementation of work-hour limits and systemic improvements. *The Joint Commission Journal on Quality and Patient Safety, 33*(11):19–29.

     Creating a Just Culture

Langley, G. J., Nolan, K. M., Nolan, T. W., Norman, C. L. & Provost, L. P. (1996). *The Improvement Guide.* San Francisco: Jossey-Bass.

Leggat, S. G. (2007). Effective healthcare teams require effective team members: defining teamwork competencies. *BMC Health Services Research, 7*(17):1–10.

Lindrooth, R. C., Bazzoli, G. J., Needleman, J. & Hasnain-Wynia, R. (2006). The effect of changes in hospital reimbursement on nurse staffing decisions as safety net and nonsafety net hospitals. *Health Services Research, 41*(3):701–720.

Lorenz, S. G. (2008). 12-hour shifts. An ethical dilemma for the nurse executive. *Journal of Nursing Administration, 38*(6):297–301.

MacPhee, M., Espezel, H., Clauson, M. & Gustovson, K. (2009). A collaborative model to introduce quality and safety content into undergraduate nursing leadership curriculum. *Journal of Nursing Care Quality, 24*(1):83–89.

Marquis, B. L. & Huston, C. J. (2006). *Leadership Roles and Management Functions in Nursing: Theory and Application,* 5th ed. Philadelphia: Lippincott Williams & Wilkins.

Mastal, M. F., Joshi, M. & Schulke, K. (2007). Nursing leadership: Championing quality and patient safety in the boardroom. *Nursing Economics, 25*(6):323–330.

McClatchey, S. (2001). Disease management as a performance improvement strategy. *Topics in Health Information Management, 22*(2):15–23.

McKeon, L. M., Oswaks, J. D. & Cunningham, P. D. (2006). Safeguarding patients. Complexity science, high reliability organizations, and implications for team training in healthcare. *Clinical Nurse Specialist, 20*(6):298–304.

Montgomery, K. L. (2010). Is it time to pull the plug on 12-hour shifts? Part 1. Barriers to change and executive leadership strategies. *Journal of Nursing Administration, 40*(4):147–149.

Moroney, N. & Knowles, C. (2006). Innovation and teamwork: Introducing multidisciplinary team ward rounds. *Nursing Management, 13*(1):28–31.

National Quality Forum (NQF). (2010). *Safe Practices for Better Healthcare—2010 Update: A Consensus Report.* Washington, DC: NQF.

Nieva, V. F. & Sorra, J. (2003). Safety culture assessment: A tool for improving patient safety in healthcare organizations. *Quality and Safety in Health Care, 12*(6):1–7.

Norris, B. (2009). Human factors and safe patient care. *Journal of Nursing Management, 17*:203–211.

Page, A., ed. *Keeping Patients Safe: Transforming the work environment of nurses.* Washington, DC: National Academies Press; 2004.

Perow, L. & Williams, S. (2003). Silence. *Harvard Business Review, 81*(5):52–58.

Perry, S. J. (2004). An overlooked alliance: Using human factors engineering to reduce patient harm. *Joint Commission Journal on Quality and Safety, 30*(8):455–459.

Pravikoff, D. S., Tanner, A. B. & Pierce, S. T. (2005). Readiness of U.S. nurses for evidence-based practice. *American Journal of Nursing, 105*(9):40–51.

Pronovost, P. J. & Goeschel, C. A. (2010). Viewing health care delivery as science: Challenges, benefits, and policy implications. *Health Services Research, 45*(5):1–15.

Pronovost, P., Holzmueller, C. G., Needham, D. M., Sexton, J. B., Miller, M., Berenholtz, S., Wu, A. W., Perl, T. M., Davis, R., Baker, D., Winner, L. & Morlock, L. (2006). How will we know patients are safer? An organization-wide approach to measuring and improving safety. *Critical Care Medicine, 34*(7):1988–1995.

Pronovost, P. & Sexton, B. (2005). Assessing safety culture: guidelines and recommendations. *Quality and Safety Health care*, *14*:231–233.

Pronovost, P., Weast, B., Holzmueller, C. G., Rosenstein, B. J., Kidwell, R. P., Haller, K. B., Sexton, J. B. & Rubin, H. R. (2003). Evaluation of the culture of safety: Survey of clinicians and managers in an academic medical center. *Quality and Safety in Health Care*, *12*:405–410.

Pronovost, P., Weast, B., Rosenstein, B., Sexton, J. B., Holzmueller, C. G., Paine, L., Davis, R. & Rubin, H. R. (2005). Implementing and validating a comprehensive unit-based safety program. *Journal of Patient Safety*, *1*(1):33–40.

Redding, D. A. & Robinson, S. (2009). Interruptions and geographic challenges to nurses' cognitive workload. *Journal of Nursing Care Quality*, *24*(3):194–200.

Richman, J. & Mercer, D. (2004). Modern language or spin? Nursing newspeak and organizational culture: New health scriptures. *Journal of Nursing Management*, *12*:290–298.

Riley, W. (2009). High reliability and implications for nurse leaders. *Journal of Nursing Management*, *17*:238–246.

Rivard, P. E., Rosen, A. K. & Carroll, J. S. (2006). Enhancing patient safety through organizational learning: Are patient safety indicators a step in the right direction? *Health Services Research*, *41*(4):1633–1653.

Rogers, A. E., Hwang, W., Scott, L. D., Aiken, L. H. & Dinges, D. F. (2004). The working hours of hospital nurses and patient safety. *Health Affairs*, *23*(4):202–212.

Romano, P. S., Geppert, J. J., Davies, S., Miller, M. R., Elixhauser, A. & McDonald, K. M. (2003). A national profile of patient safety in U.S. hospitals. *Health Affairs*, *22*(2):154–166.

Rose, J. S., Thomas, C. S., Tersigni, A., Sexton, J. B. & Pryor, D. (2006). A leadership framework for culture change in health care. *The Joint Commission Journal on Quality and Patient Safety*, *32*(8):433–442.

Rozich, J. D., Howard, R. J., Justeson, J. M., Macken, P. D., Lindsay, M. E. & Resar, R. K. (2004). Standardization as a mechanism to improve safety in health care. *The Joint Commission Journal on Quality and Safety*, *30*(1):5–14.

Ruchlin, H. S. (2004). The role of leadership in instilling a culture of safety: Lessons from the literature. *Journal of Healthcare Management*, *49*(1):47–58.

Safeek, Y. & May, P. T. (2010). Protocols, prompters, bundles, checklists, and triggers: Synopsis of a preventable mortality reduction strategy. *Physician Executive* (March/April):22–26.

Salmon, M. (2007). Care quality and safety: Same old? *Nursing Outlook*, *55*(3):117–119.

Sammer, C. E., Lykens, K., Singh, K. P., Mains, D. A. & Lackan, N. A. (2010). What is patient safety culture? A review of the literature. *Journal of Nursing Scholarship*, *42*(2):156–165.

Scott, I. (2009). What are the most effective strategies for improving quality and safety of health care? *Internal Medicine Journal*, *39*:389–400.

Scott, L. D., Rogers, A. E., Hwang, W. & Zhang, Y. (2006). Effects of critical care nurses' work hours on vigilance and patients' safety. *American Journal of Critical Care*, *15*(1):30–37.

Sheridan-Leos, N. (2008). Oncology care setting design and planning part I: Concepts for the oncology nurse that improve patient safety. *Critical Journal of Oncology Nursing*, *12*(2):361–363.

Sherwood, G. & Drenkard, K. (2007). Quality and safety curricula in nursing education: Matching practice realities. *Nursing Outlook*, *55*(3):151–155. Doi: 10.1016/j.outlook.2007.02.004.

 Creating a Just Culture

Shojania, K. G. & Grimshaw, J. M. (2005). Evidence-based quality improvement: The state of the science. *Health Affairs, 24*(1):138–150.

Shteyenberg, G., Sexton, B. J. & Thomas, E. J. (2005). *Test Retest Reliability of the Safety Climate Scale. Technical Report 01-05.* The University of Texas Center of Excellence for Patient safety Research and Practice (AHRQ grant # 1P01HS1154401 and U18HS116401). Retrieved from *www.uth.tmc.edu/schools/med/imed/patient_safety/questionnaires/SAQBibliography.html* on October 28, 2010.

Singer, S., Meterko, M., Baker, L., Gaba, D. M, Falwell, A. & Rosen, A. (2007). Workforce perceptions of hospital safety culture: Development and validation of the patient safety climate in healthcare organizations survey. *Health Services Research, 42*(5):1999–2011.

Singer, S., Dunham., Bowen., J. D., Geppert, J. J., Gaba, D. M., McDonald, K. M. & Baker, L. C. (2005). Lessons in safety climate and safety practices from a California hospital consortium. Advances in Patient Safety, 3:411–423.

Singh, H. & Vij, M. S. (2010). Eight recommendations for policies for communicating abnormal test results. *The Joint Commission Journal on Quality and Patient Safety, 36*(5):226–232.

Smith, E. L., Cronenwett, L. & Sherwood, G. (2007). Current assessments of quality and safety education in nursing. *Nursing Outlook, 55*(3):132–137.

Snoby, P. (2004). Performance improvement bootcamp. *Journal of Radiology Nursing, 23*:68–77.

Sorra, J. S. & Nieva, V. F. (2004). Hospital survey on patient safety culture. *AHRQ Publication No. 04-0041.* Rockville, MD: Agency for Healthcare Research and Quality.

Spath, P. L., ed. (2000). *Error Reduction in Health Care: A Systems Approach to Improving Patient Safety.* San Francisco: Jossey-Bass.

Spath, P. L. (2002). Don't let the human factors derail "best practices". *Outcomes Management, 6*(1):4–9.

Sportsman, S. (2010). Staffing and scheduling. In: Yoder-Wise, P. *Leading and Managing in Nursing 5ᵗʰ ed.* St Louis: Elsevier.

Stanton, M. W. & Rutherford, M. (2004). Hospital nurse staffing and quality of care. *Research in Action, 14* (AHRQ Pub. No. 04-0029). Rockville MD: Agency for Healthcare Research and Quality.

Stichler, J. F. (2010). Evaluating the evidence in evidence-based design. *Journal of Nursing Administration, 40*(9):348–351.

Stone, P. W., Mooney-Kane, C., Larson, E. L., Horan, T., Glance, L. G., Zwanziger, J. & Dick, A. W. (2007). Nurse working conditions and patient safety outcomes. *Medical Care, 45*(6):571–578.

Surani, S. & Murphy, J. (2007). Sleepy nurses. Are we willing to accept the challenge today? *Nursing Administration Quarterly, 31*(2):146–151.

Tamuz, M. & Harrison, M. I. (2006). Improving patient safety in hospitals: Contributions of high reliability theory and normal accident theory. *Health Services Research, 41*(4):1654–1676.

Ting, H. H., Shojania, K. G., Montori, V. M. & Bradley, E. H. (2009). Quality improvement science and action. *Circulation, 119*:1962–1974.

Tucker, A. L. & Spear, S. J. (2006). Operational failures and interruptions in hospital nursing. *Health Services Research, 41*(3): 643–662.

Unruh, L. Y. & Fottler, M. D. (2005). Patient turnover and nursing staff adequacy. *Health Services Research, 41*(2):599–612.

Vazirani, S., Hays, R. D., Shapiro, M. F. & Cowan, M. (2005). Effect of a multidisciplinary intervention on communication and collaboration among physicians and nurses. *American Journal of Critical Care, 14*(1):71–77.

Vera, A. & Kuntz, L. (2007). Process-based organization design and hospital efficiency. *Health Care Management Review, 32*(1):56–65.

Wachter, R. M. (2004). The end of the beginning: Patient safety five years after "to err is human." *Health Affairs,*W4:534–545.

Wachter, R. M. & Pronovost, P. J. (2009). Balancing "no blame" with accountability in patient safety. *The New England Journal of Medicine, 361*(14):1401–1406.

Wakefield, A., Attree, M., Braidman, I., Carlisle, C., Johnson, M. & Cooke, H. (2005). Patient safety: Do nursing and medical curricula address this theme? *Nurse Education Today, 25*:333–340.

Weick, K. E. (1987). Organizational culture as a source of high reliability. *California Management Review, 29*(2):112–126.

Weingart, S. N., Farbstein, K., Davis, R. B. & Phillips, R. S. (2004). Using a multihospital survey to examine the safety culture. *The Joint Commission Journal on Quality and Safety, 30*(3):125–132.

Wilkins, A. (1983). The culture audit: A tool for understanding organizations. *Organizational Dynamics, 12*(2):24–38.

Yates, G. R., Hochman, R. F., Sayles, S. M. & Stockmeier, C. A. (2004). Sentara Norkolk General Hospital: Accelerating improvement by focusing on building a culture of safety. *The Joint Commission Journal on Quality and Safety, 30*(10):534–542.

Yates, G. R., Bernd, D. L., Sayles, S. M., Stockmeier, C. A., Burke, G. & Merti, G. E. (2005). Building and sustaining a systemwide culture of safety. *The Joint Commission Journal on Quality and Patient Safety, 31*(12):684–689.

Yoder-Wise, P. (2010). *Leading and Managing in Nursing,* 5th ed. St. Louis: Elsevier.

References

1. Health and Safety Commission Advisory Committee on the Safety of Nuclear Installation, 1993.

2. Kaissi, A. (2006). An organizational approach to understanding patient safety and medical errors. *Health Services Research, 25*(4):292–305.

3. Akins, R.B., Cole, B.R. (2005). Barriers to implementation of patient safety systems in healthcare institutions: Leadership and policy implications. *The Journal of Patient Safety,* 1(1).

4. Pronovost, P. & Sexton, B. (2005). Assessing safety culture: guidelines and recommendations. *Quality and Safety Health Care,* 14:231–233.

   Creating a Just Culture

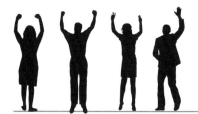

Nursing Education
Instructional Guide

Target Audience

- Nurse managers

- Ancillary managers

- Chief nursing officers

- Directors of nursing

- VPs of nursing

- Staff development specialists

- Clinical nurse leaders

- Advanced practice nurses

- Quality improvement specialists

- Human resource specialists

Statement of Need

This 150-page handbook will provide strategies for nurse leaders to implement a just and safe culture within their healthcare organizations. It will teach the history of just culture in healthcare, nursing's role in a just culture, and steps toward creating a just culture within a particular facility. This guide also provides information for adverse and near-miss event reporting, culture surveying, and implementing quality improvement efforts.

Educational Objectives

Upon completion of this activity, participants should be able to

- Describe a just culture

- Identify why reporting errors is a critical component patient safety

- Recognize barriers to error reporting

- Recognize the differences between human error, at-risk behavior, and reckless behavior

- Define culture

- Identify ways to assess organizational culture

- Select strategies to identify stakeholders and champions

- State learning objectives for a staff just culture educational program

- Describe the important of near-miss reporting

- Identify strategies for streamlining error reporting

- Name implementation steps to a just and safe culture

- Identify positive tactics for supporting a safe and just culture

- Select the types of data that should be reviewed in order to support a safe and just culture.

- Recall which steps should be taken for continuous evaluation of a safe culture

- Recognize proven strategies from other hospitals for successful safe and just culture implementation

- Identify cultural barriers to appropriate disclosure

- Identify who should disclose an error

- Identify useful techniques for improvement science

- Identify the necessary skill set for a nurse manager to adequately assist in implementing a just culture

- Recognize steps nurse managers should take to successfully assist in implementing a just culture

Faculty

Vivian B. Miller, BA, CPHQ, LHRM, CPHRM, FASHRM, has more than 25 years of progressive consultative and managerial experience in professional liability claims, patient safety, quality, and risk management services within the insurance and healthcare delivery industries. Miller is senior risk management specialist for the American Society for Healthcare Risk Management (ASHRM), serving as the internal staff resource on healthcare management content. Her personal knowledge, research and a professional network enhances the range and quality of ASHRM offerings. She identifies and develops risk management content to use as the basis for ASHRM programs, products and services; serves as an internal content consultant in the development of strategy initiatives, educational programs, communications campaigns, and other products and services, leading advocacy efforts; and serves as a risk management content resource to members and other constituents.

Terry L. Jones, RN, PhD, is an assistant professor of nursing in the Department of Nursing Administration and Healthcare Systems at the University of Texas at Austin School of Nursing. Jones previously served as director of care management and interim vice president of nursing administration and chief nursing officer at Parkland Health & Hospital System in Dallas. She has been published nationally and has also presented nationally on various nursing topics.

Continuing Education

Nursing contact hours

HCPro, Inc., is accredited as a provider of continuing nursing education by the American Nurses Credentialing Center's Commission on Accreditation.

This educational activity for 3 nursing contact hours is provided by HCPro, Inc.

Faculty Disclosure Statement

HCPro, Inc., has confirmed that none of the faculty, contributors, or planners have any relevant financial relationships to disclose related to the content of this educational activity.

Disclosure of Unlabeled Use

This educational activity may contain discussion of published and/or investigational uses of agents that are not indicated by the FDA. HCPro, Inc., does not recommend the use of any agent outside of the labeled indications. The opinions expressed in the educational activity are those of the faculty and do not necessarily represent the views of HCPro, Inc. Please refer to the official prescribing information for each product for discussion of approved indications, contraindications, and warnings.

Non-Endorsement of Products

Accreditation of this educational program does not imply endorsement by the ANCC or HCPro, Inc., of any products displayed in conjunction with this activity.

Instructions

In order to be eligible to receive your nursing contact hours or physician continuing education credits for this activity, you are required to do the following:

1. Read the book, *Creating a Just Culture: A Nurse Leader's Guide*

2. Complete the exam and receive a passing score of 80% or higher

3. Complete the evaluation

4. Provide your contact information on the exam and evaluation

5. Submit the exam and evaluation to HCPro, Inc.

Please provide all of the information requested above and mail or fax your completed exam, program evaluation, and contact information to

HCPro, Inc.
Attention: Continuing Education Manager
P.O. Box 3049
Peabody, MA 01960
Fax: 781/639-7857

NOTE:

This book and associated exam are intended for individual use only. If you would like to provide this continuing education exam to other members of your nursing or physician staff, please contact our customer service department at 877/727-1728 to place your order. The exam fee schedule is as follows:

Exam Quantity	Fee
1	$0
2–25	$15 per person
26–50	$12 per person
51–100	$8 per person
101+	$5 per person

Continuing Education Exam

Name: _____

Title: _____

Facility Name: _____

Address: _____

Address: _____

City: _____   State: _____   Zip: _____

Phone Number: _____   Fax Number: _____

E-mail: _____

Date Completed: _____

1. Which of the following is an example of just culture?

    a.   A nurse fails to speak up about a possible error during surgery because he feels it is not his place to correct the surgeon.

    b.   A nurse accidentally gives an overdose to a patient and reports it. An investigation is performed to determine whether systematic problems contributed to the error.

    c.   A nurse accidentally almost gives a patient an overdose of medicine, but catches her mistake and keeps it to herself out of fear of punishment.

    d.   A nurse accidentally gives an overdose to a patient, reports it, and is immediately punished. No further review of the incident is conducted.

2. Why is the reporting of errors critical to patient safety?

    a.   Reporting helps identify who made the mistake, and then organizations will know whom to punish

    b.   Once errors are reported, systematic flaws can be identified and fixed to help prevent the same errors from occurring in the future

    c.   Reporting helps human resources identify clinicians who never make a mistake

    d.   Reporting errors is not critical to patient safety

Creating a Just Culture

3. **Which of the following is a barrier to error reporting?**

   a. Ability of staff members to see their organization improve over time

   b. A leadership team that actively encourages reporting

   c. An organization in the generative or learning phase of culture in which failures are evaluated for systemic issues

   d. Individual staff members' fear of punishment for admitting an error

4. **What is at-risk behavior?**

   a. An action that shows an individual consciously chose to disregard a substantial and unjustifiable risk

   b. An inadvertent action of doing other than what should have been done, such as a slip or a mistake

   c. An action that increases risk where either the risk isn't recognized or is believed to be justified, even when it is known to be the wrong action to take

   d. An action performed under the influence of drugs or alcohol

5. **Culture is:**

   a. A static, instinctive, unchanging behavior

   b. A system of faith and worship of a deity

   c. A set of language, values, customs, and aesthetics of an individual or a group of people

   d. A set of values dependent upon ethnicity

6. **Which of the following is one way to assess organizational culture?**

   a. Conduct in-person focus groups

   b. Train new employees

   c. Survey leadership

   d. Report errors to your state

7. **Which of the following staff members would be the best candidate to be a patient safety champion?**

    a. Someone who is committed to promoting patient safety and preventing patient harm, doesn't get discouraged easily, and is flexible

    b. Someone who is constantly overwhelmed and gets upset when things change

    c. A new employee still learning the ropes

    d. Anyone who is not a frontline staff member

8. **Which of the following are learning objectives to implement into a just culture educational program?**

    a. Ensuring staff understand that they will never be punished for an error

    b. Ensuring staff understand that making mistakes is okay

    c. Ensuring staff understand the human factors associated with errors, and the kind of environment most conducive to error occurrence and prevention

    d. Ensuring staff report errors but not near misses

9. **Is near-miss reporting important to patient safety?**

    a. Yes, it's an important way for managers to know who makes the most mistakes

    b. Yes, it's an important way to reveal systematic errors that are likely to contribute to an error in the future

    c. No, near misses do not affect the patient and therefore are not important to report

    d. No, near-miss reporting increases patient harm

10. **Which of the following is the best strategy to encourage error reporting?**

    a. Make the process of reporting an error as easy and quick as possible

    b. Keep patient outcomes of errors reported confidential and do not share with staff

    c. When educating staff, be vague about the purpose of error reporting

    d. Teach staff that it is a necessary component of compliance

     Creating a Just Culture

11. **Which of the following involve steps to implement a just and safe culture?**

    a. Gain leadership buy-in, create a patient safety culture committee, and assess the current culture

    b. Gain leadership buy-in, perform a mock tracer in each unit, and rewrite every policy

    c. Survey patients, perform a mock tracer in each unit, assess the current culture

    d. Provide education to new employees only, rewrite every policy, and perform a mock tracer in each unit

12. **Which of the following is a positive tactic for supporting a safe and just culture?**

    a. The continued existence of silos (an environment that keeps departments and units separately and lacks cohesiveness)

    b. Varying disciplinary measures across units

    c. Manager resistance

    d. Structured and routine meetings for the patient safety culture committee

13. **Which of the following types of data should be reviewed in order to support a safe and just culture?**

    a. Only mistakes that caused patient deaths

    b. Mistakes that were caught before causing patient harm and ones that caused harm or death

    c. Only mistakes that caused any type of patient harm

    d. Only mistakes that are disclosed to the patient and/or family

14. **Which of the following is a step for continuous evaluation of a safe culture?**

    a. Requiring only frontline nurses on patient safety committees

    b. Making patient safety an agenda item at every board meeting

    c. Sharing event data with only leadership

    d. Terminating employees who were involved in any sort of error

15. **What is one strategy Medical City Dallas Hospital used to reinvigorate their just culture?**

    a. Keeping communication about adverse events to a minimum

    b. Excluding frontline staff from the analysis of adverse events

    c. Communicating to staff that under no circumstances will they be held accountable for errors

    d. Presenting real-life examples to the staff to demonstrate how easily adverse events can occur

16. **Which of the following is a cultural barrier to appropriate disclosure?**

    a. The patient and/or family's first language is different from the provider's first language

    b. The mistake was a systematic error

    c. The patient is upset

    d. The hospital has no protocol for disclosing errors

17. **Who should disclose an error?**

    a. The CEO only

    b. Risk management only

    c. The responsible licensed independent practitioner or his or her designee should take the lead in disclosing the error

    d. The legal department only

18. **Which of the following is one technique for improvement science?**

    a. Process mapping

    b. Patient rounds

    c. Mock tracers

    d. Disclosing errors

19. **Which of the following is part of a necessary skill set for a nurse manager to adequately assist in implementing a just culture?**

    a. A master's degree

    b. A master's in business administration

    c. A knowledge of the science of safety

    d. At least five years of managerial experience

20. **Fill in the blank: It is important that the nurse manager engage in _____ to clarify his or her beliefs and values about patient safety before making a commitment to participate in any cultural transformation initiatives.**

    a. Reflective thinking

    b. Patient rounds

    c. Orientation

    d. A punitive culture

 Creating a Just Culture

Continuing Education Exam Answer Key

(Please record all exam and evaluation answers here)

Name: _____   License #: _____

Facility: _____   Title: _____

Address: _____

City: _____   State: _____   ZIP: _____

Phone: _____   E-mail: _____

(Certificates are e-mailed to learners unless otherwise stated here)

Please record the letter of the correct answer to the corresponding exam question below:				
1.	5.	9.	13.	17.
2.	6.	10.	14.	18.
3.	7.	11.	15.	19.
4.	8.	12.	16.	20.

Continuing Education Evaluation

1 = Strongly Agree	2 = Agree	3 = Disagree	4 = Strongly Disagree

(Please rate the responses below according to the scale above to rate the quality of this educational activity)

1.   Please indicate how well you feel this activity met the learning objectives listed: 1   2   3   4

2.   Objectives were related to the overall purpose/goal of the activity: 1   2   3   4

3.   This activity was related to my continuing education needs: 1   2   3   4

4.   The exam for the activity was an accurate test of the knowledge gained: 1   2   3   4

5.   The activity avoided commercial bias or influence: 1   2   3   4

6.   This activity met my expectations: 1   2   3   4

7.   The format was an appropriate method for delivery of the content for this activity: 1   2   3   4

8.   Will this activity enhance your professional practice?   Yes   No

9.   How much time did it take for you to complete this activity? _____

10. Do you have any additional comments on this activity? _____
_____

Return completed form to:
HCPro, Inc. • Attention: Continuing Education Manager • P.O. Box 3049, Peabody, MA 01960 •
Telephone: 877/727-1728 • Fax: 781/639-7857

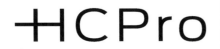